Pocket Examiner

Therapeutics

Zachary Johnson
MRCPI MFCMI DTM&H DCH

Alexander Lawrence
MB ChB MRCP(UK)

Pitman

PITMAN PUBLISHING LIMITED
128 Long Acre, London WC2E 9AN

A Longman Group Company

First published 1985

Library of Congress Cataloging in Publication Data

Johnson, Zachary.
  Pocket examiner in therapeutics.

  Companion v. to: Pocket examiner in medicine/
Alexander Lawrence.
  Includes index.
  1. Therapeutics— –Handbooks, manuals, etc.
I. Lawrence, Alexander. II. Lawrence, Alexander.
Pocket examiner in medicine. III. Title. [DNLM:
1. Therapeutics— –examination questions. WB 18 J71p]
RM104.J65 1985   615.5'076   85–6271
ISBN 0 272 79706 5 (pbk.)

British Library Cataloguing in Publication Data

Johnson, Zachary
  Pocket examiner in therapeutics.
  1. Pathology – Problems, exercises, etc.
  I. Title II. Lawrence, Alexander
  616'.0076   RB119

ISBN 0-272-79839-8

Printed at The Bath Press, Avon

Contents

Preface

This book is intended to help medical students preparing for examinations in therapeutics and medicine. At a time when the number and variety of medical textbooks seems to be growing exponentially the student can find himself having to read, digest and memorize a bewildering morass of material. It is necessary for him to extract certain important pieces of information of practical value in order to pass his examinations and, more importantly, to begin to function usefully as a doctor. While there are no short-cuts to reading the textbook, *Pocket Examiner in Therapeutics* aims to assist the busy student by highlighting important facts in a way which aids recall.

Both questions and answers contain factual information as this was the format used in our companion volume *Pocket Examiner in Medicine*, which was enthusiastically received. However, in the present book we have aimed for higher taxonomic levels and have included more questions set in a clinical context. We have also included a table of reference values for therapeutic drug monitoring as this has become an important aspect of modern therapeutics.

The book should prove useful both to students studying and revising on their own and to those working in groups. The detailed index should be of value when time is short, especially when preparing for the oral or 'viva' examination.

We hope it will help all our readers to get the best out of the efforts they have put into reading and studying therapeutics.

ZJ
AL

Acknowledgements

We would like to thank Anne Coogan, Miriam King, Deirdre Linehan, Doreen Smith and Gillian Sullivan, all of whom typed various sections of the book.
A major debt of gratitude is owed to our wives and families who had to endure many late nights during the preparation of *Pocket Examiner in Therapeutics*.

List of Abbreviations

ACTH	Adrenocorticotrophic hormone
ADH	Antidiuretic hormone
AIDS	Acquired immunodeficiency syndrome
ANA	Antinuclear antibody
AV	Atrioventricular
β–HCG	β human chorionic gonadotrophin
CNS	Central nervous system
CSF	Cerebrospinal fluid
CVP	Central venous pressure
DC	Direct current
DIC	Disseminated intravascular coagulopathy
ECG	Electrocardiogram
ENT	Ear, nose and throat
ESR	Erythrocyte sedimentation rate
FDP	Fibrin degradation products
GIT	Gastrointestinal tract
G6PD	Glucose–6–phosphate dehydrogenase
GUT	Genitourinary tract
HLA	Human leucocyte antigen
HTIG	Human tetanus immunoglobulin
HUS	Haemolytic uraemic syndrome
ICU	Intensive care unit
IM	Intramuscular
IMV	Intermittent mandatory ventilation
ITP	Idiopathic thrombocytopenic purpura
IU	International units
IV	Intravenous
K^+	Potassium ion
KCl	Potassium chloride
LDH	Lactic dehydrogenase
LVEDP	Left ventricular end-diastolic pressure
mCi	Millicuries
$MgSO_4$	Magnesium sulphate
Na^+	Sodium ion
NaCl	Sodium chloride
$NaHCO_3$	Sodium bicarbonate
NIDDM	Non-insulin dependent diabetes mellitus
NSAID	Non-steroidal anti-inflammatory drug
NSU	Non-specific urethritis
PAN	Polyarteritis nodosa
PCV	Packed cell volume

PD	Peritoneal dialysis
PRV	Polycythaemia rubra vera
PT	Prothrombin time
PTT	Partial thromboplastin time
PUVA	Psoralens and long-wave ultraviolet light
RBBB	Right bundle-branch block
SA	Sinoatrial
SC	Subcutaneously
SIADH	Syndrome of inappropriate anti-diuretic hormone
SLE	Systemic lupus erythematosus
TCT	Thrombin clotting time
TSH	Thyroid-stimulating hormone
TTP	Thrombotic thrombocytopenic purpura

1 Questions

Cardiovascular Disorders

Angina pectoris

1   Beta blockers, of which propranolol is the best established, slow the heart rate (negative chronotropic effect) and reduce the rate of muscle-fibre shortening. Myocardial oxygen consumption is reduced and beta blockers are therefore an effective treatment for angina.

Under what cardiac conditions may it be dangerous to give beta blockers?

2   Sublingual glyceryl trinitrate is absorbed rapidly and causes venous and arteriolar dilatation within 2 minutes. The effect lasts 20 to 30 minutes. Isosorbide dinitrate is absorbed from the GI tract and has a longer duration of action.

The vasodilatation produced by nitrites and organic nitrates commonly causes throbbing headaches. How can these headaches be managed?

3   Nitroglycerin is absorbed through the skin and is available and moderately effective in a graduated-release transcutaneous preparation.

What is the effect of nitrites and nitrates on haemoglobin?

4   Amylnitrite by inhalation is an alternative to sublingual nitroglycerin but it is less effective.

What effect do the nitrites and organic nitrates have on heart rate and heart size?

5   Nifedipine, a calcium channel blocker, is a coronary as well as a peripheral vasodilator and is the drug of choice in Prinzmetal variant angina, which is due to coronary artery spasm. It is also frequently effective in exertional angina.

How does one determine the correct dose of this drug?

Myocardial infarction

6   In the initial phases of acute myocardial infarction, treatment for heart failure and arrhythmias may be necessary.
      What other treatment should be given routinely?

7   The pain of myocardial infarction is typically severe and distressing and effective doses of potent analgesics are an important part of management. Morphine and diamorphine are often used with a small dose of prochlorperazine to counteract nausea.
      A patient with an extensive infarction and hypotension is given morphine 20 mg IM. What is wrong with this therapy?

8   The left ventricle tolerates increases in volume poorly and when its function is impaired, as in acute myocardial infarction, it is important to avoid excessive fluid administration.
      An IV line is necessary, however, during the first few days of an acute infarction to provide immediate access for the treatment of arrhythmias. What fluid would you use and at what rate?

9   In acute myocardial infarction, hypotension may be due to excessive vasodilator therapy, dehydration from profuse sweating, or more commonly from pump failure due to left ventricular myocardial damage. Only in this last instance is it appropriate to give dopamine or dobutamine.
      What is the dose of dopamine and how would you regulate it?

10   Diabetic control is frequently upset by myocardial infarction. For the first few days it may be necessary to use a sliding scale or a continuous low-dose infusion of insulin.
      What useful effects does insulin have in acute myocardial infarction apart from controlling blood glucose?

11   In right ventricular infarction, which may be
      present to some degree in up to a third of in-
      ferior infarctions, the clinical sign of a raised
      jugular venous pressure is not an indication for
      diuretic therapy.
         Assuming that Swan–Ganz catheter pressure
      measurements meet all the criteria for right
      ventricular infarction what is the correct fluid
      management?

12   Complications of a pulmonary artery flotation
      catheter (often called a Swan–Ganz catheter)
      are uncommon but may include pulmonary in-
      farction and pulmonary embolism.
         How may the risk of these two complications
      be minimized?

13   On admission for acute anterior wall myocardial
      infarction a patient's ECG shows complete right
      bundle-branch block with a normal axis. During
      the first night the QRS complexes on the moni-
      tor change their amplitude and a further ECG
      shows that the axis has changed to –45°.
         What does the change of axis indicate and
      what is the correct management of this develop-
      ment?

14   In the technique of intra-aortic balloon counter-
      pulsation, inflation of the balloon is syn-
      chronized with early diastole and deflation with
      early systole.
         How does this help coronary artery flow?

15   In cardiac arrest external cardiac massage is
      essential and a 2–inch depression of the
      sternum is desirable. It has been widely believed
      that this is effective because the heart is being
      squeezed.
         What is a more plausible explanation?

16   Anticoagulation reduces the incidence of venous
      and arterial thromboembolism in patients with
      myocardial infarction. Patients who are especi-
      ally vulnerable to thromboembolic complic-
      ations are those with congestive cardiac failure,
      hypotension, a history of thromboembolism
      and a large infarction.
         Low-dose subcutaneous heparin is often used
      for prophylaxis against venous thrombosis and
      pulmonary embolism. What is the dose?

17   Although it has become common to mobilize
      patients who are free of complications in the
      first few days after myocardial infarction, it
      has recently been shown that early mobilization
      increases the incidence of left ventricular ab-
      normalities when patients have been assessed 2
      or more years after the infarction.
         How long should patients with acute myo-
      cardial infarction stay in hospital?

18   Following myocardial infarction, coronary
      artery bypass surgery improves survival in
      patients with a high risk of reinfarction.
         Which coronary angiographic findings
      identify the high–risk group to whom surgery
      should be offered?

19   Patients who survive a myocardial infarction are
      at an increased risk of further infarction when
      compared with the general population. Correc-
      tion of risk factors is logical but of uncertain
      benefit once infarction has already occurred.
         Apart from surgery (coronary artery bypass
      grafting) which drugs may possibly reduce the
      incidence of reinfarction?

20   When a patient is discharged from hospital after
      a myocardial infarction clear advice is important
      in order to give the patient confidence as well
      as the best chance of fitness. Smoking must
      stop and obesity be avoided.
         What advice would you give regarding:

      (a)   exercise,
      (b)   sexual intercourse,
      (c)   return to work?

21   Patients with heart disease are at increased
      risk under general anaesthesia. Pre-anaesthesia
      risk factors include hypertension, a gallop
      rhythm and atrial or ventricular extrasystoles.
         Following a myocardial infarction how long
      should general anaesthesia be postponed,
      ideally?

Congestive cardiac failure

22   In congestive cardiac failure, digoxin has been
      one of the traditional mainstays of treatment.
      In recent years, however, the use of digoxin for

patients in sinus rhythm has been increasingly
questioned.
   Why is this?

23   Digoxin administered IV begins to act within an
     hour. Oral digoxin is absorbed relatively quick-
     ly and peak plasma levels are reached within
     an hour, but onset of action is somewhat later.
        What haemodynamic changes may occur in
     the first 20 minutes following IV administration
     which are unrelated to the drug's long-term
     positive inotropic effect?

24   The absorption of digoxin taken orally may be
     reduced by concurrent consumption of choles-
     tyramine or foods containing a large quantity
     of bran.
        How long does it take for a dose of digoxin
     to be distributed in all the body tissue?

25   A patient on digoxin for congestive cardiac fail-
     ure develops digoxin toxicity soon after being
     started on quinidine for troublesome extra-
     systoles.
        Why should digoxin toxicity have developed?

26   The commonest cause of digoxin toxicity is
     potassium depletion resulting from simultaneous
     treatment with thiazide or loop diuretics.
        In what other circumstances may digoxin
     toxicity occur?

27   A patient taking digoxin and spironolactone
     develops gynaecomastia and complains of head-
     aches and abdominal discomfort.
        Which drug is the likely cause of these side
     effects?

28   In patients with severe congestive cardiac failure
     large doses of diuretics may lead to hypona-
     traemia and azotaemia.
        Apart from vasodilators, which alternative or
     supplementary therapy can be effective without
     causing volume depletion and reduced renal
     perfusion?

29   Potassium depletion is an ever-present risk of
     diuretic therapy with thiazides, frusemide and
     related drugs in congestive cardiac failure (and
     other states associated with secondary hyper-
     aldosteronism). Patients who forget to take

their potassium supplements or cannot tolerate them are especially at risk.

What are the therapeutic alternatives to these diuretics?

30 A patient treated with frusemide once daily for congestive cardiac failure complains that the diuresis in the ensuing 4 hours after the dose is extremely inconvenient.

What alternative can you offer?

31 Soon after starting treatment for congestive cardiac failure, a diabetic patient notices that his urine contains more sugar than usual while another patient develops an attack of gout. A third patient comes with a rash affecting face and hands.

Which drug used to treat congestive cardiac failure could be the cause of these events?

32 In the treatment of congestive cardiac failure, diuretics are traditionally used to overcome fluid retention due to secondary hyperaldosteronism. By themselves, however, diuretics do not alter cardiac function very much unless there is a reduction in circulating fluid volume and with it a reduction in venous return to the heart.

Which group of drugs act haemodynamically to improve cardiac function, resulting in a diuresis?

33 Potent diuretics such as frusemide or bumetanide are urgently indicated by the IV route in the treatment of acute pulmonary oedema. These drugs have a weak vasodilator effect but principally act by reducing circulating volume and lowering venous return to the heart.

What other method is there for achieving the same result?

34 A 55 year old insulin-dependent diabetic lady with chronic renal failure is admitted in pulmonary oedema with a blood pressure of 160/120. Her antihypertensive therapy has previously consisted of a small dose of methyldopa.

Apart from the fact that her treatment has been inadequate, which sort of drug would be more suitable to treat both her hypertension and left ventricular failure?

35   In congestive cardiac failure secondary hyper-
      aldosteronism and renal underperfusion both
      operate to conserve sodium, leading to a net
      retention of sodium. It is therefore logical to
      restrict dietary sodium.
          In which situation may it be appropriate to
      administer sodium to patients with treated
      congestive cardiac failure?

Cardiac arrhythmias

36   In atrial fibrillation, digoxin is used to slow the
      ventricular rate. This is the only application of
      digoxin which is not in dispute.
          Which drugs may be combined with digoxin
      to give a more regular ventricular rate than that
      produced by digoxin alone?

37   In atrial fibrillation, digoxin is useful for slow-
      ing the ventricular rate. In this situation it is
      safe to use digoxin because it is possible to
      observe and adjust the therapeutic effect easily.
      If the arrhythmia is of recent onset, digoxin
      may restore sinus rhythm. Sinus rhythm can
      also be restored with DC cardioversion.
          Which drug may be useful in maintaining
      sinus rhythm after atrial fibrillation has been
      converted?

38   Paroxysmal supraventricular tachycardias may
      be due to a re-entry mechanism if an accessory
      pathway is present, as in the Wolff–Parkinson–
      White syndrome.
          Which drug is often effective in blocking the
      accessory pathway during an attack?

39   The paroxysmal supraventricular tachycardias
      of Wolff–Parkinson–White syndrome may
      seriously interfere with normal life if frequent,
      prolonged and unresponsive to drug therapy.
          What further help may be offered to the
      patient?

40   In the acute stages of myocardial infarction,
      particularly inferior infarction, sinus brady-
      cardia is a relatively common arrhythmia. It
      is important to correct it, especially if there is
      any fall in blood pressure.
          What is the first drug to use?

41   When atropine fails to correct sinus bradycardia
      in acute myocardial infarction the next drug to
      try is isoprenaline. The best way to give it is by
      IV infusion, titrating the dose against the heart
      rate.
           In making up the IV solution what quantities
      of isoprenaline and fluid are used?

42   For ventricular extrasystoles and ventricular
      tachycardia complicating myocardial infarction
      or acute ischaemia, lignocaine is the first drug
      to use. It is customary to give an IV bolus
      followed by a continuous infusion.
           What doses should be used?

43   A patient on a lignocaine drip complains of
      dizziness and double vision. These are recog-
      nized side effects of lignocaine. If the dose is
      not reduced or the drug withdrawn, convulsions
      may ensue.
           Can lignocaine cause a fall in blood pressure?

44   Mexiletine has an action similar to lignocaine in
      suppression of ventricular arrhythmias following
      acute myocardial infarction. It can be given IV
      or orally.
           In which respect does it differ from ligno-
      caine?

45   In many hands disopyramide has replaced
      procainamide for the oral maintenance therapy
      of ventricular arrhythmias. The average daily
      requirement is 600 mg divided into three or
      four doses.
           Why may male patients find this drug unsuit-
      able?

46   Procainamide is still used for the suppression of
      ventricular extrasystoles and tachycardias, both
      as IV therapy during the acute stages of myo-
      cardial infarction and as oral maintenance
      therapy subsequently.
           How long is its half-life and how frequently
      should it be administered?

47   When episodes of ventricular tachycardia con-
      tinue to occur in acute myocardial infarction
      despite full doses of lignocaine, procainamide,
      mexiletine or disopyramide, which drug may
      still be effective?

48 If patients with paroxysmal or sustained atrial or ventricular tachyarrhythmias do not respond to beta blockers, disopyramide, quinidine, procainamide, mexiletine or digoxin, which drug may be effective?

In view of its effectiveness in this difficult therapeutic situation why is it not a first–line drug?

49 Potassium, which should be administered cautiously, is the first line of therapy in digoxin cardiotoxicity. DC shock carries a significant risk in the presence of digitalization.

Which drugs can be used to treat digoxin-induced ventricular arrhythmias?

50 An idioventricular rhythm occurs when a ventricular focus discharges at a faster rate than the SA or AV nodes but not fast enough to be classed as a ventricular tachycardia, i.e. less than 100 beats per minute.

In the setting of acute myocardial infarction how should idioventricular rhythms be treated?

51 Digitalization is the only contraindication to DC cardioversion which is otherwise generally a safe and effective treatment for atrial or ventricular arrhythmias.

How should the patient be prepared and which drugs should one have ready to give after the shock?

52 Following myocardial infarction, Mobitz type II AV block and bifascicular block may both precede complete heart block.

Which prophylactic measure should be undertaken to prepare for the development of complete heart block?

53 Some arrhythmias can be due to unwanted effects of antiarrhythmic drugs and correct therapy may be to withdraw medication.

Which antiarrhythmic drugs, apart from digoxin, can cause AV block?

Hypertension

54 An overweight, middle-aged man is found to be hypertensive when attending his general practitioner for an insurance examination. His blood pressure is 160/110.

What steps should be taken and what advice given before any drugs are prescribed?

55   If weight loss, increased exercise, avoidance of stress and restriction of salt fail to improve mild hypertension (or are impracticable), drug treatment is probably advisable, although the benefits of drug treatment for mild hypertension have been disputed.

   Thiazide diuretics are commonly chosen for initial therapy. How do they reduce blood pressure?

56   Although studies of potassium losses during thiazide therapy for hypertension have indicated that potassium supplements should not be necessary, the fact that potassium-sparing diuretics have a similar antihypertensive action without the risk of potassium depletion gives them considerable therapeutic value.

   Why are thiazides still so widely used?

57   Although there are convincing epidemiological observations linking a population's average blood pressure to its salt intake, it is often not clear that an individual's salt intake at the time his hypertension is detected, usually in adult life, is important. It is possible that adult hypertension represents a homeostatic setting determined by exposure to salt much earlier in life.

   Nevertheless hypertensives are generally advised to restrict their salt intake. Which recent experimental findings give credence to this old piece of advice?

58   In the initial treatment of mild to moderate hypertension, beta blockers are widely used. In a patient with hypertension exacerbated by emotion or a fast heart rate they are particularly appropriate.

   How do beta blockers lower blood pressure?

59   Both cardioselective and non-cardioselective beta blockers are effective in the treatment of hypertension.

   In which rare form of hypertension will beta blockers tend to aggravate the condition?

60   When a beta blocker alone fails to correct hypertension the addition of a diuretic is often effective in controlling moderate hypertension. For

more severe hypertension, hydralazine is a better drug to add.

Apart from the fact that hydralazine is a more potent antihypertensive agent, why is beta blocker plus hydralazine a successful combination?

61   When hypertension is not controlled by a single drug, a second drug should be added. Some drug combinations are more logical and effective than others.

What is the rationale for adding spironolactone to a thiazide?

62   When hypertension remains severe in spite of full doses of beta blockers, vasodilators and diuretics, minoxidil or captopril can be tried. Minoxidil is a vasodilator and must be given with a beta blocker and a diuretic. It hardly ever fails to control hypertension but fluid retention must be anticipated and hirsutism is invariable.

How does captopril work?

63   Alpha-methyldopa is usually effective for controlling mild to moderate hypertension but it is being used less now that other drugs are available.

What are the negative attributes of alpha-methyldopa?

64   When antihypertensive treatment with one drug fails, an alternative to adding a second preparation is to try a more potent drug on its own. Two drugs which were effective but have gone out of fashion are reserpine (a cause of depression) and guanethidine, a ganglion blocker which causes significant drug interactions.

Prazosin, however, is a reasonably well tolerated antihypertensive drug and is often effective on its own. How should prazosin therapy be initiated?

65   When a combination of two drugs fails to control hypertension, it is customary to add a third drug. A common combination is beta blocker plus vasodilator plus diuretic, but drugs may be used which have more than one action. Examples are labetalol and indapamide, the latter being a thiazide derivative with a marked vasodilator action.

Would you use the commercially available preparations containing two or three drugs in a single tablet instead of prescribing the drugs individually?

66   Clonidine is an antihypertensive agent that
works by blocking central synapse alpha receptors. It is often effective as single drug therapy
in mild to moderate hypertension and, since the
dose is small (0.2–0.8 mg per day in divided
doses), it does not interfere with urinary assays
for catecholamines.

     What is the main precaution to observe with
clonidine?

67   The commonest reason for hypertension to remain uncontrolled in the face of full therapy is
non-compliance. Non-compliance often continues when the gravity of severe hypertension
has been repeatedly explained.

     How should such exasperating patients be
managed?

68   In some people with hypertension it is possible
to identify an aetiological factor related to a
driving and intolerant personality. Blood
pressure may be normal or only a little raised
on rising but is considerably higher at the end
of a day's work. Mild sedation may be an effective part of the therapy, e.g. diazepam 2 mg
twice daily.

     In what other way may such people manage
to control their blood pressure?

69   In the treatment of hypertension it must not
be overlooked that restoration of blood pressure to what is considered 'normal' may lead
to deterioration in renal function, angina, confusion or worsening claudication.

     Why is this?

70   Blood pressure is commonly measured in the
lying position but it is important to measure it
standing also since the finding of postural hypotension is a significant physical sign.

     What does postural hypotension indicate?

71   In malignant hypertension, blood pressure
will often respond to hydralazine (20 mg IM) or
nifedipine (20 mg sublingually), both drugs usually achieving a smooth reduction of pressure to
safe levels.

     How quickly does the blood pressure respond
to these two forms of therapy?

72   When faced with hypertensive encephalopathy

and a need to reduce blood pressure to safe levels rapidly, the therapeutic choice lies between a sodium nitroprusside infusion, parenteral hydralazine, sublingual nifedipine or IV diazoxide.

How is diazoxide given and why is this drug falling out of favour?

73 Sodium nitroprusside by continuous IV infusion is a very effective way to lower high blood pressure rapidly. While the pressure is being controlled other therapy must be started so that the pressure remains at a safe level when sodium nitroprusside is withdrawn.

Why should sodium nitoprusside be used with caution in renal failure and which routine test indicates cyanide toxicity?

74 Although secondary hypertension is relatively uncommon it should be looked for since it offers the chance of a cure in many cases. The finding of hypokalaemia in a patient who has not received diuretics is the best clue to the presence of adrenal disease.

Which drugs should one specifically enquire about when looking for secondary hypertension?

75 Renal artery stenosis is one of the commonest potentially correctable causes of hypertension. The results of surgery are unpredictable, however, and cases of doubtful operability are better treated medically.

Which new technique may offer a more effective alternative to surgery?

Rheumatic carditis

76 In rheumatic carditis salicylates are the drugs of choice to control the symptoms. In severe cases, however, headache, nausea and tinnitus may occur before an adequate blood level is obtained.

What alternative therapy can be offered in this situation?

Bacterial endocarditis

77 In patients with prosthetic valves or rheumatic heart disease antibiotic prophylaxis is very im-

portant before minor surgical procedures in order to prevent bacteraemia which may lead to endocarditis. For dental or ENT procedures, procaine penicillin 1.2 megaunits should be given IM 30–60 minutes before the procedure. Alternatively oral phenoxymethyl penicillin 500 mg every 6 hours can be given with the procedure being scheduled 1 hour after the second dose. In GUT (e.g. cystoscopy), GIT and biliary tract procedures the pathogens are different.

Which antibiotics should be used for prophylaxis in these situations?

78   In the antibiotic prophylaxis of patients with prosthetic heart valves or rheumatic heart disease, penicillin is recommended for dental and ENT procedures while ampicillin plus gentamicin is recommended for GUT, GIT or biliary tract procedures.

Which antibiotics should be used for patients allergic to the penicillins?

79   The antibiotic treatment of infective endocarditis depends both on the type of organism and on the organism's sensitivity to antibiotics as measured by bacterial growth in serial dilutions of the treated patient's serum.

What is the usual first choice of treatment for *Streptococcus faecalis* endocarditis?

80   *Staphylococcus epidermidis* is a common pathogen in infective endocarditis. It is usually not very virulent but it is very difficult to eradicate. If the organism is fully sensitive to benzylpenicillin, 24–40 megaunits IV daily for 6–8 weeks is the recommended therapy.

Which antibiotics should be considered if the organism is resistant to benzylpenicillin?

Pericardial disease

81   Pericarditis is a common complication of myocardial infarction in the first few days and the pain usually responds to either aspirin or paracetamol. Dressler's syndrome, of which pericarditis is the most constant feature, is less common but often requires more than simple analgesics.

Which drugs are used?

82   When pericardial fluid causes cardiac tamponade, ventricular filling in diastole is impeded.

Any measures which reduce venous return and ventricular filling, e.g. diuretic therapy, should be avoided. Removal of pericardial fluid is a matter of urgency if the patient is deteriorating. If closed pericardiocentesis is decided on, arrangements should also be made for surgery in case the closed procedure is unsuccessful.

What are the three least dangerous sites for inserting the needle in closed pericardiocentesis?

Dissecting aneurysm

83   In acute dissecting aneurysm of the aorta immediate therapy of any hypertension is indicated. What is needed is a rapid but short-acting agent which can be given by continuous IV infusion permitting finger-tip control of the systolic blood pressure to 100–120 mmHg. In addition the drug should reduce cardiac output.

Which antihypertensive agent meets these requirements and is the drug of choice?

Thromboembolic disease

84   In pulmonary thromboembolism, IV heparin is commonly the drug of first choice (except when the clinical condition is critical and facilities for administering streptokinase are available). Heparin is usually given as a loading dose followed by a continuous infusion regulated by a pump.

How would you calculate the dose?

85   After initiation of anticoagulant therapy in pulmonary thromboembolic disease with heparin it is customary to change to an oral anticoagulant such as warfarin for maintenance therapy. Pharmacokinetic drug interactions with warfarin are extremely important since too little or too much anticoagulant effect may be disastrous.

In which ways do drugs interfere with warfarin?

86   In several studies streptokinase has been shown to give much better short- and long-term results than heparin in the treatment of pulmonary embolism and deep vein thrombosis. There is considerable hesitation in using it, however, as

there is some evidence that it carries a greater
risk of haemorrhage than heparin.

What are the two undisputed contraindications to using streptokinase and what is
the usual dose?

Respiratory Disorders

Bacterial pneumonia

87   In bacterial pneumonia, as in any infection, the
choice of antibiotic, the route of administration
and the size of the dose is decided on the basis
of the suspected pathogen, the condition of
the patient and the presence of any underlying
diseases likely to adversely affect recovery. A
seriously ill patient with an upper lobe pneumonia is treated with 2 megaunits of benzylpenicillin IV every 4 hours until cultures reveal
the presence of *Klebsiella pneumoniae*.

How should the antibiotics be changed?

88   Confirmation of a diagnosis of Legionnaire's
disease may take several days due to the
necessity either to culture the organism on
special media or in a guinea pig, or to demon-
strate a rising antibody to *L. pneumophila* in
paired sera by an indirect immunofluorescent
method. Occasionally it may be possible to
identify the organism in a bronchial or tracheal
aspirate by immunofluorescence.

Pending results of these tests, how should a
case of suspected Legionnaire's disease be
managed?

Pleurisy

89   The pain and inflammation of viral pericarditis
and pleurisy may both respond to NSAIDs.
What is the usual dose of indomethacin and
what side effects are common?

Atypical pneumonia

90   Atypical pneumonias may be due to
Mycoplasma pneumoniae, *Chlamydia psittaci*
or *Coxiella burneti*.

To which antibiotic are these organisms sensitive and what alternative is there in the case of *Mycoplasma*?

Pulmonary tuberculosis

91   Pyrazinamide and ethionamide are two bacteriostatic antituberculous drugs, both of which may cause nausea and vomiting and drug-induced hepatitis.
      What effect does pyrazinamide have on uric acid?

92   Isoniazid and rifampicin are the only two antituberculous drugs which are bactericidal. In slow acetylators isoniazid commonly causes a peripheral neuropathy which is reversible with pyridoxine (vitamin B6). Hepatitis is fortunately an uncommon side effect because it is usually very serious when it occurs.
      What are the side effects of rifampicin? What important drug interactions may occur with rifampicin?

93   Chemoprophylaxis against tuberculosis may be considered in contacts with a strongly positive tuberculin test, but without clinical or radiological evidence of tuberculosis. However, age, likelihood of recent infection and ethnic group influence the decision on chemoprophylaxis.
      What chemotherapeutic regime is normally prescribed for tuberculosis chemoprophylaxis?

Asthma

94   Salbutamol is a selective β_2 receptor agonist. When administered by aerosol inhalation, either from a pressurized 'puffer' or a nebulizer, onset of action is rapid and side effects are less than with systemic therapy.
      What is the adult dose by inhalation and what are the side effects of salbutamol?

95   Salbutamol, the most selective β_2 agonist, can be given in place of aminophylline in the treatment of asthma. An IV injection of 250 μg every 4 hours or a continuous infusion of 3–20 μg/min may be used.

In which other situation may IV salbutamol be helpful?

96 Non-selective beta blockers such as propranolol block both β_1 and β_2 receptors. In patients with asthma beta blockers will tend to cause bronchospasm. The risk of bronchospasm is less with blockers selective for β_1 receptors.
    Name three cardioselective beta blockers.

97 Aminophylline is a bronchodilator used in asthma and left ventricular failure. It is administered IV or orally (in sustained release forms). Rapid IV injection (in less than 5–10 minutes) causes cardiac arrhythmias and even arrest.
    What is the usual dose for IV administration?

98 Aminophylline in excess causes tremor and tachycardia and occasionally convulsions. The therapeutic plasma level lies between 30 and 80 μmol/l.
    What factors affecting the drug's half-life must be taken into account when deciding on a patient's dose?

99 Adrenaline (epinephrine) stimulates both α and β_1 and β_2 adreno-receptors. In the lungs β_2 stimulation is predominant leading to bronchodilation. Adrenaline is usually effective in the early stages of an attack of asthma.
    What is the usual dose and route of administration for an adult?

100 If acute attacks of asthma do not respond to combined therapy with β_2 agonists (salbutamol) and phosphodiesterase inhibitors (aminophylline), it is essential to give steroids without delay. Hydrocortisone 200 mg (or 4 mg/kg) every 4 hours is the usual adult treatment, changing to a reducing course of oral prednisone when the patient is well enough to swallow oral medications.
    When asthma is sufficiently severe to warrant maintenance therapy with steroids, what are the alternatives to oral prednisone and what is their main side effect?

101 Sodium cromoglycate stabilizes mast cell membranes, blocking release of histamine in re-

sponse to IgE binding. It has no place in the treatment of an established attack of asthma or rhinitis.

In which types of asthma is it effective? What is the normal starting dose?

102 Antihistamines are much less effective than bronchodilators and cromoglycate in the treatment and prevention of asthma, but occasionally they may be useful. In nocturnal asthma due to allergy to house dust mites in the bedroom, a mild prophylactic effect may combine with mild sedation to give uninterrupted sleep.

What is the usual dose of chlorpheniramine?

103 The ideal way to prevent attacks of atopic asthma is to avoid exposure to the allergen(s).

What advice would you give in this regard to a patient with house dust allergy?

104 Exercise-induced asthma can be prevented by taking medication prior to exercise.

Which medications are effective?

105 Some patients with extrinsic asthma and allergic rhinitis are helped by courses of desensitizing injections. The ingredient antigens of the injections are based on the most positive reactions in skin tests.

How are the injections given for a patient with pollen allergy?

Chronic bronchitis and emphysema

106 Early initiation of antibiotic treatment is an important aspect of therapy of acute exacerbations of chronic bronchitis, most of which are due to *Haemophilus influenzae* or *Streptococcus pneumoniae*. To this end the patient should have a supply of antibiotics at home.

Which antibiotics should he use?

107 In some patients with chronic bronchitis, acute exacerbations are very frequent and there may be a case for continuous low-dose antibiotic therapy, e.g. cotrimoxazole two tablets daily.

What is likely to happen with this form of therapy?

108 There is a non-infective component to the chronic inflammation and irritation associated with mucus-secreting gland hypertrophy in chronic bronchitis. This may explain why some patients with chronic bronchitis benefit from systemic steroids.

What dose is usually given?

109 Pulmonary hypertension is a common sequel to chronic lung disease and may also follow repeated pulmonary emboli or occur as a primary disease in young women. Hydralazine, prazosin, aminophylline and isoprenaline may each relax pulmonary vascular smooth muscle and effect a reduction in pressure.

What is the safe limit to the daily dosage of hydralazine and how could you tell that it was effective?

110 Influenza vaccine is of limited value since the vaccine may not contain the antigens of the prevalent strain of virus. Nevertheless, it is reasonable to vaccinate those at high risk, namely chronic bronchitics, the elderly and those living in institutions.

Why must allergy to eggs be excluded before the vaccine is given?

111 The many techniques for giving up smoking include acupuncture, hypnosis, group therapy, complete inhalation of successive cigarettes to the point of nausea, exposure to full medical illustration of cancer and other smoking-related diseases and the use of nicotine-containing chewing gum.

Which method has the lowest relapse rate?

Respiratory failure

112 When carbon dioxide retention develops in chronic lung disease, the respiratory centre relies on hypoxia for stimulation. Administration of too much oxygen will correct hypoxia but respiratory drive will be diminished. This then results in further accumulation of CO_2.

How much oxygen should be given in respiratory failure and how does one adjust the dose for each patient?

113 Strong analgesia is often withheld from patients

with chronic respiratory failure in the belief that morphine and related drugs will cause serious depression of respiration.

Why is this practice erroneous?

114 Patients with endoctracheal tubes cannot cough effectively and are therefore vulnerable to retained secretions. Regular endotracheal tube suction is a vital part of the routine care of an intubated patient.

Which precaution in performing suction helps to reduce the incidence of nosocomial chest infection?

115 Respiratory stimulants such as nikethamide and doxapram have little clinical application. They may be useful, however, in staving off terminal respiratory failure in a patient who is no longer considered a candidate for mechanical ventilation.

How is doxapram given?

116 It is dangerous to have a patient on mechanical ventilation who is either paralysed or completely sedated.

Why is this, and what is a preferable arrangement?

117 On a volume-cycled ventilator (in contrast to a pressure-cycled ventilator) one can set the tidal volume. The gas flow rate determines the speed at which the tidal volume is delivered and the proportion of each respiratory cycle taken up with inspiration.

What is the desirable inspiration/expiration ratio when ventilating an asthmatic patient?

118 In primary hypoventilation a small, but clinically useful, improvement may be obtained with medroxyprogesterone.

What is the principle behind the use of a progestogen in this situation?

Lung neoplasms

119 The most effective cough suppressants are also drugs of addiction, namely, morphine, diamorphine and codeine. All cause constipation as a side effect.

Under what circumstances is it reasonable to use these drugs in a cough linctus?

120 Small cell carcinoma of the lung is regarded as
a systemic disease. By the time the condition
is diagnosed, the tumour has seeded in many
different parts of the body.
      What bearing does this have on treatment
of this condition?

121 Complete resection of a non-metastatic tumour
offers the only certain chance of cure in lung
cancer.
      In which situation would you advise patients
with lung cancer to undergo surgery?

Pulmonary sarcoidosis

122 In progressive pulmonary sarcoidosis, treatment
with corticosteroids is indicated.
      For how long is it necessary to continue
treatment?

Respiratory physiotherapy

123 In patients with abdominal surgical wounds,
peritoneal dialysis or other reasons for limited
inspiration, incentive spirometry is a useful
method for maintaining tidal volume and
preventing basal atelectasis.
      Which forms of chest physiotherapy are use-
ful for patients with retained sputum?

Alveolitis

124 Allergic alveolitis may remit spontaneously
following removal of the patient from exposure
to the offending antigenic dust.
      How should patients be managed whose
signs and symptoms persist despite withdrawal
of the offending antigen?

125 In fibrosing alveolitis the only treatment which
may affect the usually downhill progression of
the disease is steroid therapy.
      How successful is steroid therapy?

Bronchoscopy

126 Bronchoscopy is a diagnostic technique for

obtaining a tissue diagnosis in diseases of the bronchi and lung parenchyma.

What are the therapeutic applications of bronchoscopy?

Pneumothorax

127 If a pneumothorax is large enough to cause dyspnoea, a chest drain with an underwater seal should be inserted.

How would you decide when it is safe to remove the drain?

Gastrointestinal Disorders

Hiatus hernia

128 The symptoms of hiatus hernia are usually relieved by regular antacid therapy, weight reduction, small meals and avoidance of stooping. Raising the head of the bed is also important. A satisfactory method is to place a brick under each leg of the bed.

If these measures fail what may be present?

Peptic ulceration

129 In addition to medication, what advice should you give patients with peptic ulcers?

130 Tri-potassium di-citrato bismuthate has a success rate in the healing of duodenal ulcers similar to that of cimetidine. It is given in courses of 28 days.

What is its mode of action?

131 Metoclopramide stimulates gastric emptying while at the same time relaxing the pylorus and duodenal bulb. This may explain why it can give symptomatic relief in some cases of dyspepsia. Its antiemetic action may also be valuable.

What is carbenoxolone and what is its most important side effect?

132 Cimetidine and ranitidine block H_2 histamine receptors in the stomach leading to approxi-

mately 50% and 70% reduction in acid production respectively. This action has a beneficial effect on ulcer healing but gastric acid production returns to pretreatment levels as soon as treatment is discontinued.

What precautions must be exercised in the follow-up of gastric ulcers treated with these drugs?

133 To heal peptic ulcers it has been shown that cimetidine and ranitidine can be given in divided daily doses or as a single bedtime dose for 4–6 weeks. Thereafter, continuation of the bedtime dose helps prevent relapse.

What side effects can cimetidine cause?

134 Antacids are popular remedies in the occasional treatment of dyspeptic symptoms. They also have an important place in the treatment of established peptic ulceration. Their neutralizing power varies between preparations, however, and in many cases is inadequate to give more than a few minutes rise is gastric pH.

What dose of antacid would be expected to give the best chance of curing a duodenal ulcer?

135 Antacids should not be taken at the same time as other medications because of interference with drug absorption.

To which commonly prescribed drugs does this particularly apply?

136 In the management of dyspepsia and peptic ulcer disease bland diets have gone out of fashion in favour of either high-fibre diets or low-fat diets. Many patients merely avoid a few isolated items of food.

Should food be given to a patient with upper gastrointestinal bleeding?

137 Milk has a traditional place in the diet of a peptic ulcer patient, but the reason for this is not clear. Some patients may actually experience hyperacidity after milk, and elimination of dairy products can often bring relief from chronic dyspepsia.

Which constituent of milk stimulates gastrin production?

138 Cimetidine slightly reduces portal venous flow

and inhibits the P450 cytochrome oxidase system. This may explain its interactions with a large number of other drugs whose pharmacokinetics are influenced by hepatic metabolism.

Which commonly used drugs are metabolized more slowly when given with cimetidine?

Gall bladder disease

139 Chenodeoxycholic acid is a bile salt administered therapeutically to dissolve pure cholesterol gall stones. Dissolution occurs very slowly, so that treatment may need to continue for up to 2 years. It should not be used when the gall bladder is not functioning.

What is the main side effect of chenodeoxycholic acid?

140 In acute cholecystitis, non-surgical treatment consists of rest, IV fluids, analgesia and antibiotics. It is felt that there is an advantage in using antibiotics which enter the bile in therapeutic levels.

Which antibiotics qualify in this respect?

Portal hypertension

141 When portal hypertension and hypoalbuminaemia lead to ascites, secondary hyperaldosteronism develops and there is a rise in body sodium. This further contributes to ascites. In this situation restriction of dietary sodium to less than 22 mEq per day is very important. Diuretics are used to remove ascites but weight loss should not exceed 0.7–0.9 kg per day.

Why is this?

142 Therapeutic paracentesis to relieve the discomfort of tense ascites is seldom necessary (in contrast to diagnostic paracentesis which is virtually always indicated). Cannula insertion may cause bowel perforation or bleeding from the puncture of a blood vessel.

What complications may follow removal of the fluid?

Oesophageal varices

143 In the initial treatment of bleeding oesophageal
varices, the dose of vasopressin is 20 units in
100 cc of 5% dextrose over 10 minutes IV.
   How long does the effect of this dose last
and what might make you suspect that the
vasopressin was inert?

144 When IV vasopressin fails to control bleeding
from oesophageal varices the next step is to
use a Sengstaken–Blakemore tube. When the
tube is in place, the head of the bed should be
elevated to minimize the risk of inhaling
oesophageal blood or secretions coming from
above the oesophageal balloon.
   What volume of air should be injected into
the gastric balloon and to what pressure should
the oesophageal balloon be inflated?

Malabsorption

145 Adherence to a gluten-free diet gives remission
in nearly 90% of cases of coeliac disease and
improvement in many cases of dermatitis
herpetiformis.
   What medications may be necessary in
coeliac disease, at least in the early stages of
treatment?

146 In bacterial overgrowth of the small intestine
(due to bowel surgery etc.), tetracyclines may
be the antibiotic of choice.
   What treatment regimen would you use?

Drug absorption

147 The presence of food in the stomach and small
intestine can influence all aspects of drug pharmacokinetics, but the greatest effect is on drug
absorption. With frusemide and bumetanide,
for instance, food will delay absorption. The
same dose is ultimately absorbed but the
diuretic effect is extended over a longer period.
   What effect does the presence of food have
on the absorption of iron, rifampicin, isoniazid
and levodopa?

Inflammatory bowel disorders

148 In ulcerative colitis sulphasalazine in a daily
dose of up to 4 g will relieve a mild attack and
help prevent relapses. It is usually given long
term. In the presence of G6PD deficiency it
may cause haemolysis.
    What is the action of sulphasalazine on
Crohn's disease (regional enteritis)?

149 Prednisolone is of major importance in severe
attacks of both ulcerative colitis and Crohn's
disease. For maintaining a remission, however, its usefulness is limited to ulcerative
colitis. There is no evidence of benefit in this
respect in Crohn's disease.
    What is the place of azathioprine in the
treatment of inflammatory bowel disease?

150 Ulcerative proctitis, a mild form of ulcerative
colitis in which the inflammation is confined
to the rectum, can be treated successfully with
topical steroids.
    In what form can the steroids be given and
what is the dose? What treatment should be
used if topical steroids fail?

151 Sodium cromoglycate, which inhibits mast cell
degranulation, has been found to be effective in
some cases of ulcerative colitis when taken
orally.
    In which other intestinal condition can it be
effective?

Diarrhoea

152 Codeine and phenoxylate are common remedies
for diarrhoea. They work by slowing transit
time and allowing more water absorption. Their
use is not advisable in infective diarrhoeas.
    What other drug is effective for diarrhoea
and for controlling ileostomy flow without the
risk of developing drug dependence? What is
the usual adult daily dose?

Constipation

153 Diets containing little fibre can result in both
chronic constipation or chronic diarrhoea, due

to abnormal water content in the stool. The remedy lies in introducing fibre which helps to return the stools to normal consistency. This in turn has a beneficial effect on the functional disturbances of bowel mobility known as the irritable bowel syndrome.

What preparations contain fibre?

154 Bisacodyl, danthron, phenolphthalein and senna are all stimulant laxatives which increase intestinal motility within 6–8 hours of ingestion. In chronic laxative abuse it is these drugs which are commonly taken in great excess, resulting in a non-functioning colon and hypokalaemia.

Which urine test reveals the consumption of phenolphthalein?

155 Enemas, usually phosphate enemas, are commonly given for severe constipation resistant to laxatives given orally or rectally. They may be given also prior to surgical procedures, although in the case of sigmoidoscopy their use may give a false impression of mucosal irritation.

In which situation is a magnesium sulphate enema a valuable and urgent therapy?

156 Di-octyl sodium succinate is a stool softener and relieves constipation by making the stools easier to pass.

In which clinical situations is it desirable to avoid straining at stool?

Abdominal sepsis

157 The use of prophylactic antibiotics is no substitute for strict asepsis and careful surgery in the prevention of postoperative abdominal sepsis. However, judicious use of antibiotics active against the likely pathogens may be of value in some situations.

Can you suggest a reasonable prophylactic regime for a major colorectal operation?

Liver and Pancreatic Disorders

Hepatic encephalopathy

158 Hepatic encephalopathy can be precipitated
by infection, constipation, sedation or
hypokalaemia.
   Which drugs are liable to cause or aggravate
hypokalaemia?

159 Phenothiazines are potentially hazardous in the
presence of liver disease, not only because
hepatotoxicity is one of their side effects but
also because their sedative properties may
precipitate hepatic encephalopathy.
   Which antiemetic would you prescribe in
liver disease?

160 Sedation is contraindicated in hepatic failure
because of the danger of aggravating
encephalopathy. In the event of a patient
being dangerously restless (pulling out IV
lines or nasogastric tube or fighting to get out
of bed), many would advocate the use of
phenobarbitone (60 mg IM).
   What is it about this drug's pharmacokinetics that makes it acceptable under such
difficult circumstances?

161 In hepatic encephalopathy measures to reduce
ammonia and amine absorption from the gut
include cleansing enemas ($MgSO_4$), lactulose
and oral neomycin (1 g orally every 6 hours).
   What kind of diet should be given?

162 Valine, leucine and isoleucine comprise the
branched-chain amino acids.
   What is the theoretical justification for
administering these in hepatic encephalopathy?

163 Lactulose is a synthetic disaccharide which the
gut is unable to absorb. It acts as a laxative
probably by an osmotic effect, although it
is metabolized by bacteria in the colon.
   Apart from being a laxative, what important application does lactulose have?

Viral hepatitis

164 A 15 year old schoolboy develops cholestatic jaundice following a 2-week period of nausea and anorexia. Serum transaminase levels are moderately elevated but the boy is not seriously ill. Hepatitis B surface antigen is not present in his serum, but there is a high titre of anti-hepatitis A IgM.

What is the place of diet, vitamin supplements, bed rest and steroids in his management?

165 Following accidental exposure to hepatitis B, e.g. from a needle-prick after taking blood from an HBsAg positive patient, immediate passive protection is available in the form of IM gamma-globulin. There is now a vaccine against hepatitis B.

Which groups of patients and staff are recommended to have the vaccine and what has been the theoretical objection to this vaccine?

Chronic active HBsAg negative hepatitis

166 Chronic active HBsAg negative hepatitis is the only form of liver disease for which corticosteriods are firmly indicated.

What influence do steroids have on life expectancy and the development of cirrhosis in this condition?

167 If treatment with daily prednisolone fails to bring improvement in chronic active HBsAg negative hepatitis or if side effects are severe, azathioprine can be added.

Which commonly used drug interferes with the metabolism of azathioprine?

Cholestasis

168 Cholestyramine is an anion exchange resin which binds with bile salts in the gut and leads to their faecal excretion. This depletes the body pool of bile salts, which is desirable in the treatment of the itching associated with cholestasis but it makes bile more lithogenic and interferes with the absorption of fats and fat-soluble vitamins.

What drug interactions may occur between

cholesytramine and digoxin, paracetamol and
warfarin respectively?

Drugs and liver disease

169 When prescribing the oral contraceptive pill to
women with underlying disease the risk from
the drug must be balanced against the risk from
pregnancy.
What is the place of the oral contraceptive in
patients with liver disease?

170 The presence of chronic liver disease can cause
serious problems in the treatment of tuberculosis since the two bactericidal antituberculous drugs isoniazid and rifampicin can both
cause hepatotoxicity, as can pyrazinamide,
ethionamide and para-amino salicylic acid.
Which antituberculous drugs carry a low risk
of hepatotoxicity?

171 In the presence of liver disease the metabolism
of a large number of drugs is slowed and this
may lead to increased drug effects or side
effects. Two examples of this are cimetidine,
in which a confusional state is more likely to
occur, and aminophylline, in which a normal
dose may precipitate tremor and palpitations.
Which side effects of corticosteroids and
NSAIDs are more common in the presence of
liver disease?

Wilson's disease

172 In the treatment of Wilson's disease, penicillamine is the drug of choice. It chelates copper
thus increasing urinary excretion. Treatment is
started with 300 mg four times daily and may
be increased to a total of 2 g daily if there is no
improvement after 6 months.
For how long should therapy be continued?

Pancreatic disease

173 In the treatment of acute pancreatitis the use of
pethidine, IV fluids and nasogastric suction is not
in dispute. Antibiotics are often given to prevent secondary infection. Some would advocate
giving aprotinin.

What is aprotinin and in what doses is it given IV?

174 A 5 year old child with cystic fibrosis is expected to need 1 g of pancreatin before each meal to compensate for deficient pancreatic function.
Why is it advisable to give cimetidine as well?

Renal Disorders

Glomerulonephritis

175 Experimental and clinical evidence implicating antibodies and antibodies to antibodies (the network theory) in glomerulonephritis has led to the use of cytotoxic drugs such as cyclophosphamide in conjunction with steroids.
Which side effects preclude the use of cyclophosphamide as long-term therapy?

176 In the treatment of glomerulonephritis, as in other diseases, the use of corticosteroids requires a careful balancing of desirable pharmacological effect against the numerous unwanted and occasionally serious side effects. Side effects are usually minimal with short-term therapy and with maintenance therapy of 20 mg prednisone daily or less.
Which forms of glomerulonephritis are sensitive to steroids?

177 Plasmapheresis or plasma exchange is an expensive but important technique for removing plasma protein, either because of hyperviscosity or because of the presence of pathogenic antibodies or other plasma factors.
In which diseases has it been found to be useful?

178 SLE always involves the kidneys, although in many cases this is only apparent on a renal biopsy. Biopsy-only renal involvement is not an indication for steroid therapy.
When would you give steroids with or without cytotoxic drugs?

Nephrotic syndrome

179 Renal vein thrombosis occurs in patients with nephrotic syndrome, especially children, and in association with pregnancy.

What is the treatment for renal vein thrombosis?

180 In the nephrotic syndrome it may be possible to mobilize the oedema with (initially) large doses of diuretics, e.g. chlorothiazide 2 g daily.

What alternative therapy may be effective and also improve the response to diuretics?

Renal tubular acidosis

181 In distal renal tubular acidosis, treatment to correct the acidosis is with sodium bicarbonate in adults and sodium citrate solution in children. Depending on the degree of potassium deficiency, potassium citrate can be added to sodium citrate. Up to 8 g of citrate or bicarbonate may be necessary daily.

How is the correct dose determined?

182 In patients (mostly children) with proximal renal tubular disorders, of which the commonest is cystinosis, indomethacin can bring a striking improvement in the severe symptom of polyuria.

What action does indomethacin have on the kidney that explains this effect?

Urinary tract infection

183 In urinary tract infections it has become apparent that a single dose of a bactericidal antibiotic is sufficient to eradicate lower tract infection (cystitis) in the great majority of cases. Conversely, in the case of renal parenchymal infection, some authorities recommend 6 weeks antibiotic therapy following 10 days parenteral therapy, especially if there is an underlying predisposition to infection, e.g. diabetes.

Which antibiotic best penetrates the prostate? What measures would you advise for a woman with recurrent cystitis related to sexual intercourse?

Renal Stones

184 In idiopathic hypercalciuria, oral cellulose phosphate (5 g three times daily) can reduce calcium absorption and correct the hyper-calciuria.

What alternative medication can reduce calcium excretion without affecting calcium absorption?

185 The best way to reduce urinary oxalate ex-cretion is to reduce dietary oxalate consump-tion.

Is it correct that tea, coffee, strawberries and asparagus are high in oxalate?

186 Some cases of urolithiasis in which the stones contain oxalate are due to hyperoxaluria. Hyperoxaluria may be dietary or metabolic in origin. Increased oxalate absorption is a side effect of cellulose phosphate consumption.

In primary hyperoxaluria what treatment may succeed in reducing oxalate excretion (in addition to a low oxalate diet)?

Renal artery stenosis

187 Renal artery stenosis is an uncommon but potentially correctable cause of secondary hypertension. Traditional surgical procedures include bypass grafting and renal autotrans-plantation.

What alternative, non-surgical method of treatment is more successful in specialized centres?

Renal failure

188 Sodium is a dietary and therapeutic factor whose regulation is important in renal failure. Inadequate intake can be as harmful as excess, and it is generally wise to measure output and ensure that it is matched by intake.

How many millimoles of sodium are con-tained in 1 gram of sodium chloride and sodium bicarbonate respectively?

189 Phosphate retention develops in moderately severe renal failure and increases as renal func-

tion deteriorates. Its importance lies in the reciprocal depression of calcium which contributes to renal osteodystrophy. Dietary phosphate restriction is generally impracticable given the ubiquity of phosphate.

What therapeutic alternative is there to achieve a reduction in serum phosphate levels?

190 In moderate to severe renal failure, dosages of both co-trimoxazole and ampicillin should be reduced. Co-trimoxazole should be given as two tablets daily (for adults), whereas ampicillin should be given as half the normal dose but at the same 6 hourly frequency.

What change should be made for chloramphenicol in renal failure?

191 The dosage and dose interval for many drugs require modification in renal failure. There is no simple guide to the change needed. This is because uraemia can alter pharmacokinetics in several ways. For example, a protein-bound drug may be displaced by an increased amount of free fatty acids but this reduction in protein binding may be offset by the enhancement of hepatic oxidation that occurs in uraemia.

What happens to hepatic acetylation in uraemia?

192 In the presence of renal failure there are some drugs that should not be used. Amongst them are the tetracyclines, nitrofurantoin and nalidixic acid.

Why are these drugs contraindicated in the presence of renal failure?

193 The half-life of the H_2-receptor blocker cimetidine is prolonged in renal failure and the daily dose should be halved. The antiemetic, metoclopramide, is best avoided in moderate to severe renal failure.

Why is this?

194 Digoxin and gentamicin are two drugs whose elimination is closely dependent on glomerular filtration rate. In renal failure the interval between doses must be increased or the doses reduced to allow for the greater half-life. There are formulae and tables for calculating the necessary changes, but if the patient is receiving peritoneal dialysis or haemodialysis, it becomes

almost impossible to make accurate predictions.

Under such circumstances how should the dose of the drug be regulated?

195 In chronic renal failure a normal solute load to the reduced number of functioning nephrons can often cause an osmotic diuresis and most patients with moderate to severe renal failure should have a large fluid intake. Large means 3 litres per 24 hours.

Name two other urinary tract conditions in which large fluid intake can be of therapeutic value.

196 Sodium bicarbonate is used to correct the acidosis commonly found in renal failure, distal renal tubular acidosis and following ureterocolic anastomoses.

In which non-acidotic renal diseases is sodium bicarbonate of therapeutic importance?

197 The value of protein restriction in patients with renal failure is that it protects the remaining nephrons from the damaging effect of hyper-filtration. Against restriction is the debilitating effect of under-nutrition. It is possible, how-ever, to have an effectively restricted protein diet (0.7g/kg body weight) and still consume more than the minimum daily requirement. In severe and end-stage renal failure, foods high in potassium usually need to be avoided.

Which foods are these?

198 In renal failure, 1α-hydroxylation of vitamin D precursors is impaired and there is a deficiency of 1,25-dihydroxy-vitamin D which is the most active form of the vitamin. Vitamin D therapy in renal osteodystrophy needs to be with either 1α-vitamin D or 1,25-dihydroxy-vitamin D.

In aluminium bone disease, which is un-responsive to vitamin D, which chelating agent is used to remove aluminium?

Haemodialysis

199 In chronic haemodialysis there may be a net iron loss and deficiency of water-soluble vita-mins is possible.

What is the dose of the routine adult daily supplement of iron and folic acid?

200 In haemodialysis heparinization is necessary to prevent blood clotting when it is in contact with the tubing and membranes or hollow fibres of the dialysers. Typical doses of heparin would be 2000–5000 units loading dose into the dialyser followed by 1000–2000 units hourly by an infusion pump until 1 hour before the end of dialysis.

  What refinement of heparinization can be used for patients with diabetic retinopathy and others at risk from heparin?

Peritoneal dialysis

201 Peritoneal dialysis is a relatively simple and effective way to treat renal failure. Temporary PD cannulas have no means of tissue attachment but permanent cannulas have Dacron cuffs into which fibroblasts can grow and form a watertight barrier to infection. PD can remove water very easily using hypertonic solutions, but potassium diffuses only relatively slowly.

  For which groups of patients with renal failure is chronic ambulatory PD especially preferred to haemodialysis?

Renal transplantation

202 Renal transplants require antirejection therapy for graft survival, conventionally prednisone and azathioprine. Prednisone in increased or pulse doses is effective in acute and subacute rejection, whereas for chronic rejection azathioprine is more important.

  What is the dose of prednisone and azathioprine in maintenance antirejection therapy?

203 Cyclosporin A is an antirejection drug which differs from prednisone and azathioprine in being a selective poison for differentiating lymphocytes. Following transplantation it predominantly blocks the host reaction to the graft. Renal and hepatic toxicity complicate the drug's use.

  What are the other side effects of CyA therapy?

204 Aspirin is being used in an increasing number of
conditions for its effect in impairing platelet
aggregation. Renal applications include the
treatment of chronic vascular rejection of a
transplant.
What is the ideal dose of aspirin for reducing
platelet aggregation?

Endocrine Disorders

Pituitary disorders

205 The treatment of choice for acromegaly is
microadenomectomy via the trans-sphenoidal
route in cases where the tumour is confined to
the sella turcica. This may be followed by
bromocriptine therapy if excessive growth
hormone secretion persists.
How should prolactinomas be managed?

206 Cranial diabetes insipidus should be treated
with desmopressin 10–20 μg intranasally
given sufficiently frequently to produce a
daily urine output of about 2 litres. This
usually means once or twice daily.
What factors should be considered in replacement therapy for deficiency of the anterior pituitary hormones?

207 Eighty per cent of cases of Cushing's syndrome
in adults are due to excessive ACTH production by the pituitary. The treatment of choice
is excision of the ACTH producing microad-
enoma via the trans-sphenoidal route.
In situations where pituitary surgery is not
available, or when it is not clear whether the
excessive ACTH production is pituitary or
ectopic in origin, what alternative therapy is
there?

Hyperthyroidism

208 Antithyroid drugs include carbimazole and
thiouracil derivatives and may produce sensitivity reactions such as fever, skin rashes,
arthralgia, jaundice, lymphadenopathy and
salivary gland enlargement. These reactions
are usually of short duration and may respond

to antihistamine therapy without withdrawal of the antithyroid drug.

What more dangerous toxic effect may result from antithyroid drugs?

209 Propranolol blocks the peripheral adrenergic effects of T_3 and T_4 and reduces the peripheral conversion of T_4 to T_3. However, it does not reduce thyroid hormone secretion, and its effects wear off about 6 hours after cessation of therapy.

What is the place of propranolol in the treatment of hyperthyroidism?

210 Iodide inhibits the synthesis of thyroid hormone when its concentration in the thyroid gland rises (the Wolff–Chaikoff effect). However, in hyperthyroidism this effect does not last more than about 3 weeks.

What are the indications for using iodide in the therapy of hyperthyroidism?

211 Approximately 60% of cases of Graves' disease relapse following discontinuation of antithyroid drugs. It is not possible to predict accurately which patients will remain in remission.

How should patients on antithyroid drugs be monitored?

212 Graves' disease characteristically manifests spontaneous exacerbations and remissions. The aim of drug therapy in this situation is thus to control thyroid hormone secretion until spontaneous remission occurs.

How does hyperthyroidism due to single or multiple toxic adenomas differ from this, and what are the therapeutic implications of this difference?

213 General measures used in the management of thyroid crisis include rehydration and correction of electrolyte imbalance, salicylates for hyperpyrexia and digoxin, diuretics and oxygen if cardiac failure develops. Precipitating factors such as infection should be identified and treated.

What specific treatment should be used for a thyroid crisis?

214 The first aspect of treating the ophthalmopathy of Graves' disease is to control the accompany-

ing hyperthyroidism. Symptoms due to mild exophthalmus should be treated with sunglasses, 1% methyl cellulose eye-drops and elevation of the head of the bed at night; 5% guanethidine eye-drops may also be helpful.

How should severe exophthalmus be treated?

215 Surgery is the preferred treatment in hyperthyroidism with a large goitre or obstructive symptoms. However, an important factor in deciding which treatment modality to use is the skill and experience of the surgeon.

How should thyrotoxic patients be prepared for surgery?

216 Radioiodine (^{131}I) is very useful for treating hyperthyroidism due to toxic adenomas when surgery is contraindicated or in cases of Graves' disease who have relapsed after a course of antithyroid drugs.

What problems are associated with the use of ^{131}I?

217 Hyperthyroidism in pregnancy, if not treated, can cause premature labour. Thyroid surgery may carry a similar risk if done in the first or third trimester. Thus, if indicated, it should be done in the second trimester.

What important considerations govern antithyroid drug therapy in pregnancy?

Hypothyroidism

218 The aim of therapy for hypothyroidism is to restore metabolic function to normal. The usual replacement dose of L-thyroxine is 100–200 μg/day. Adequate treatment of primary hypothyroidism is reflected by a fall of TSH levels to normal values of 8 mU/l or less.

What complications may occur when initiating treatment for hypothyroidism in elderly patients or those with underlying heart disease and what precautions should be taken in these situations?

219 Hypothyroid patients tolerate stress such as surgery or infection poorly and may develop myxoedema coma in such situations. IV therapy should be used owing to undependable absorption of drugs from the gastrointestinal

tract or muscle. 500 μg of L-thyroxine should be given immediately followed by 50–200 μg IV daily until oral therapy is possible.

What other aspects of therapy are important?

Thyroid nodules

220 Euthyroid multinodular goitres which do not have signs of malignancy should be treated with suppressive doses of L-thyroxine (200 μg/day). If the goitre progresses after 3–6 months of therapy, partial thyroidectomy should be considered.

How should the management of single thyroid nodules be approached?

Addison's disease

221 If acute hypoadrenalism is suspected, treatment should precede detailed investigation. Blood should be taken for cortisol, electrolyte and urea estimations and 100 mg of hydrocortisone should be given IV.

What additional treatment is required?

Corticosteroids

222 Administration of steroids on alternate days is an effective method of reducing the incidence of side effects of long-term steroid therapy.

How should surgery or acute medical illness be managed in patients on long-term steroids?

223 There has been considerable controversy over the question of whether or not corticosteroid therapy increases the incidence of peptic ulceration. The latest evidence suggests that steroids double the incidence of peptic ulceration from the normal population figure of 1% to 2%.

What precautions should be adopted when treating patients with long-term steroids?

Conn's syndrome

224 Approximately half of all hypertensive patients with spontaneous hypokalaemia will have primary hyperaldosteronism. Of these approximately a third will have bilateral adrenal

hyperplasia rather than an adenoma and will therefore not be candidates for surgery. Bilateral adrenal hyperplasia requires medical therapy.

What is the appropriate treatment?

Phaeochromocytoma

225 In the search for a phaeochromocytoma, the patient's medications may interfere with the diagnostic assays.

Which diagnostic test is the least vulnerable to interference and which antihypertensive drugs will not interfere with any of the diagnostic tests?

226 Preoperative management of phaeochromocytoma includes control of symptoms and hypertension with the long-acting alpha-adrenergic recepter blocker phenoxybenzamine and the alpha- and beta-receptor blocking drug labetolol.

How should these patients be managed during surgical removal of the tumour?

Hypogonadism

227 Primary androgen deficiency due to Leydig cell failure is an indication for androgen therapy. Synthetic oral androgens such as methyltestosterone can cause cholestatic jaundice and there are reports of hepatoma; thus they should not be used for long-term therapy.

How therefore should androgen deficiency be managed?

Amenorrhoea

228 Clomiphene citrate causes increased secretion of LH and FSH from the pituitary gland by blocking oestradiol receptors in the hypothalamus.

In what situations is this drug useful?

Hirsutism

229 Some mild cases of congenital adrenal hyper-

plasia may not present until after childhood.
The usual symptoms in this situation are primary amenorrhoea and hirsutism. A very good
response to dexamethasone suppression may
occur. This is an example of organic hirsutism.

What is 'dysfunctional hirsutism' and what
therapy is available for it?

Metabolic Disorders

Diabetes mellitus

230 Most diabetic patients should be treated by
some dietary modification. However, in order
to ensure a reasonable chance of patient compliance the diet prescribed must be based on
the patient's usual food habits.

Although the optimum diet for diabetics
is still under study, what proportions of carbohydrate, protein and fat would be regarded
as 'prudent' in a diabetic diet?

231 Education of the diabetic patient regarding the
nature of his disease, its management and complications is vital to ensure that he lives as
healthy a life as possible and remains free of
complications as long as possible.

Are the majority of diabetic patients
adequately informed about their condition?

232 Polydypsia and polyuria in a newly diagnosed
diabetic who is not overweight is usually
associated with significant ketonuria and is an
indication that insulin therapy is required.

What is a reasonable approach to initiation
of insulin therapy in situations where there is
no evidence of dehydration, severe hyperglycaemia or serious complications such as
ketoacidosis?

233 Mild hypoglycaemic reactions may be treated
by ingestion of a glass of milk or some carbohydrate food. Every diabetic on insulin or oral
hypoglycaemic drugs should carry some glucose
sweets or sugar lumps for use in emergencies,
but excessive use of these may produce severe
hyperglycaemia.

How should more severe hypoglycaemic reactions be managed?

234 Insulin dependent diabetic patients who are well controlled and who require elective surgery should be operated on as early in the day as possible.
How should their diabetic state be managed during and after surgery?

235 Insulin resistance is said to occur when insulin requirements exceed 200 units/days for at least 3 days. Non-immune resistance can be due to obesity, infection, ketoacidosis or various endocrine diseases.
What is the most common cause of immunologically mediated insulin resistance and how may it be managed?

236 The main indication for using sulphonylurea oral hypoglycaemic preparations is in non-insulin dependent (usually maturity onset) diabetics who are close to their ideal weight and in whom hyperglycaemia is not controlled by diet alone.
In what groups of patients should particular care be exercised in the use of these drugs?

237 Biguanides, unlike sulphonylureas, do not stimulate insulin release and therefore do not cause hypoglycaemia when used alone. They should not be used in patients with renal disease or those prone to lactic acidosis (because of cardiovascular or hepatic disease) or in alcoholics.
How do biguanides reduce blood glucose levels?

238 Careful and frequent clinical and biochemical monitoring is vital in the treatment of diabetic ketoacidosis. One of the major therapeutic priorities is correction of dehydration.
How should this be achieved?

239 Patients with diabetic ketoacidosis may have a total potassium deficit of 300–700 millimoles. Although the initial serum potassium is frequently high or normal due to the effects of acidosis, hypokalaemia is a potentially fatal complication of therapy.
How should potassium administration be managed in ketoacidosis?

240 A reasonable insulin regime for treating diabetic ketoacidosis is an initial dose of 10–20 units of short-acting insulin IM followed by 5 units per hour IM. In the presence of hypotension the insulin should be given by IV infusion.

At what stage may subcutaneous insulin be introduced?

241 Hyperosmolar non-ketotic diabetic coma is usually seen in elderly diabetics with NIDDM. The initial treatment should include administration of fluids to expand the plasma volume.

What fluid regime should be used in this situation?

242 Biochemical features of lactic acidosis include a plasma lactate of 5 mmol/l or more and an anion gap of 18 mmol/l or more. Blood sugar may be normal, elevated or low.

How should lactic acidosis in a diabetic be managed?

243 The indications for photocoagulation therapy in diabetic retinopathy are maculopathy and proliferative retinopathy.

How is the beneficial effect of photocoagulation explained?

244 Diabetes in pregnancy requires careful and skilled management because of the increased perinatal mortality in this condition. Dietary advice should aim to allow for a weight gain of 0.5 kg per week. However, vigorous restriction should be avoided in the obese.

What levels of blood glucose should be maintained in order to ensure optimum outcome for the fetus?

245 Management of diabetic patients with chronic renal failure includes tight control of hypertension and eradication of urinary tract infection. Insulin requirements fall as renal function decreases – possibly due to impaired degradation of insulin by the renal parenchyma.

Oral hypoglycaemic preparations should not be used in renal failure. Why not?

Hyperlipidaemia

246 Cholestyramine is a bile acid binding resin

which is useful for lowering plasma cholesterol in patients with hypercholesterolaemia not responsive to diet alone.

What precautions are necessary when using cholestyramine?

Inborn errors of metabolism

247 Long-term treatment of acute intermittent porphyria consists of avoiding alcohol and precipitating drugs and maintaining a carbohydrate intake of at least 300 grams per day.

Which drugs in particular should be avoided in a patient known to have acute intermittent porphyria?

248 It is well known that many drugs can precipitate an attack of acute intermittent porphyria in a genetically predisposed individual, and these should therefore be avoided in such cases.

Do you know which drugs are safe to use in cases of acute intermittent porphyria?

249 A 20 year old house painter develops severe photosensitivity during a spell of good weather. His red cell and faecal protoporphyrin levels are markedly elevated but his urinary Δ-amino laevulinic acid and porphobilinogen levels and his faecal coproporphyrin levels are normal. His father and grandfather suffered from a similar complaint.

How would you treat him?

250 In homocystinuria there is a block in the metabolism of methionine to cysteine due to cystathionine synthetase deficiency. This results in a build-up of methionine and homocystine in the plasma and homocystine in the urine.

How can homocystinuria be treated?

Disorders of Mineral and Bone Metabolism

Hypocalcaemia

251 Chronic hypocalcaemia should be managed by using calcium and vitamin D supplements.

What precautions are necessary with this treatment?

252 An acute episode of tetany may be managed effectively by the administration of 10–20 ml of 10% calcium gluconate IV.

Tetany may, however, be secondary to alkalosis. How should this be treated?

Hypercalcaemia

253 Chronic hypercalcaemia not amenable to curative measures should be controlled by a low-calcium diet, adequate hydration and phosphate supplementation.

What additional treatment may be beneficial in hypercalcaemia due to malignancy?

254 Acute hypercalcaemia should be treated by restriction of calcium intake and by vigorous rehydration with normal saline.

What other measures may be of value in this situation?

255 In chronic sarcoidosis hypercalcaemia and hypercalciuria may be present. These abnormalities will respond to steroids but cellulose phosphate, 5 g three times daily provides an alternative therapy without risk of steroid side effects.

How does it work and what disadvantages does it carry?

Disorders of phosphate and magnesium metabolism

256 Hypomagnesaemia may occur in malabsorption, alcoholism and during parenteral hyperalimentation.

In some cases convulsions may occur. How should they be managed?

257 Hypophosphataemia may occur during parenteral hyperalimentation, recovery from acidosis, recovery from starvation and in malabsorption;

How should hypophosphataemia be managed?

Metabolic bone disease

258   Nutritional osteomalacia and rickets can be
prevented by administration of 400 IU
calciferol (vitamin D_2) daily by mouth.
    How should osteomalacia secondary to
malabsorption be managed?

259   Calcitonin is an effective agent for treating
Paget's disease, but unfortunately it must be
given IM and it is usually required at least
2–3 times per week.
    Of what value are diphosphonates in the
treatment of Paget's disease?

260   Long-term administration of steroids in doses
equivalent to prednisolone 7.5 mg daily or
more is liable to lead to iatrogenic osteopenia.
    How do steroids cause this and what mea-
sures should be taken to delay or prevent it?

261   Certain general measures should be used to
delay the development of osteoporosis in post-
menopausal women. These include encourage-
ment of maximum mobility and a good dietary
intake of protein and calcium.
    Of what value are oestrogens in the pre-
vention of osteoporosis in post-menopausal
women?

Disorders of Water and Electrolyte Metabolism

Disorders of water metabolism

262   Where possible the syndrome of inappropriate
antidiuretic hormone secretion (SIADH) should
be treated by controlling the underlying cause.
This includes the withdrawal of drugs such as
chlorpropamide, phenothiazines and tricyclic
antidepressants, all of which may be associated
with SIADH.
    If this approach is unsuccessful, or not
feasible, what alternative management is
available?

263   Water intoxication occurs when excessive
quantities of water are given to patients whose
ability to excrete a water load is restricted. It
may occur in chronic renal failure, cardiac

failure, Addison's disease and cirrhosis.

A number of drugs have ADH-like effects and can cause water intoxication. What are these?

Disorders of sodium metabolism

264 Maintenance therapy for patients unable to take fluids by mouth but who do not have abnormal losses of fluid or electrolytes and who have normal renal function should provide 35 ml/kg of water, 70 mmol Na^+ (4 g NaCl), 40 mmol K^+ and 100–150 g of carbohydrates per day.

What is a reasonable IV fluid regime to prescribe in order to meet these requirements?

265 Volume depletion is usually due to loss of both sodium and water from the extracellular fluid compartment.

What precautions are necessary in treating volume depletion?

266 Sodium retention occurs when the renal excretion of sodium is less than the amount ingested. It is usually associated with water retention, thus leading to volume overload. Clinically detectable expansion of the extracellular compartment does not usually occur until it is increased by 15%.

Which drugs may cause sodium and water retention?

Disorders of potassium metabolism

267 One of the most important adverse effects of diuretic therapy is potassium depletion. This in turn may lead to digoxin toxicity. Potassium depletion may also precipitate hepatic encephalopathy in cases of hepatic failure who are treated with potent diuretics.

What is the 'low-salt syndrome' which may be associated with diuretic therapy?

268 Hypokalaemia is best treated by oral supplements. When a patient is unable to take potassium orally or when hypokalaemia is severe, parenteral potassium is required. If the serum K^+ exceeds 2.5 mmol/l and the ECG is normal,

the rate of potassium administration should not exceed 10 mmol/hour and its concentration should not exceed 30 mmol/l. Not more than 200 mmol should be given in 24 hours.

What is the maximum rate and concentration for very urgent situations?

269 Prevention of hyperkalaemia includes recognition of oliguria and avoidance of excessive ingestion of potassium supplements or potassium-sparing diuretics and limitation of dietary potassium.

How should one manage a patient with a serum K^+ of 8 mmol/l or one whose ECG shows signs of hyperkalaemia?

270 An elderly man who was taking a potassium-sparing diuretic as part of his treatment for congestive cardiac failure complains of palpitations. His ECG shows tall T waves, widened QRS complexes and almost complete loss of P waves. Hyperkalaemia is confirmed on admission to hospital.

What underlying conditions could have predisposed him to hyperkalaemia?

Acid–base disturbances

271 In a patient who is not unduly dehydrated and whose renal function is normal, metabolic acidosis of mild to moderate severity may be reversed by administration of IV normal saline alone, without any bicarbonate.

How can you explain this?

272 A 50 year old man who has been found to have severe gastric outlet obstruction due to a chronic duodenal ulcer is being prepared for surgery. His plasma bicarbonate is 40 mmol/l and blood pH is elevated.

How will you manage this biochemical problem?

273 A patient with cor pulmonale and chronic compensated respiratory acidosis is on treatment with large doses of diuretics. Following treatment of a chest infection she is found to have a persisting metabolic alkalosis, reflecting an inability to excrete accumulated bicarbonate.

How should this situation be managed?

Haematological Disorders

Aplastic anaemia

274 Chloramphenicol is a bacteriostatic antibiotic
which may cause bone marrow depression of
two types. The first type may occur in any
patient on chloramphenicol and is common in
cases with renal or hepatic impairment. Prevention of this problem is usually possible by
monitoring full blood and platelet count every
3 days in any patient on chloramphenicol and
stopping the drug at the first sign of leukopenia
or thrombocytopenia.
   What is the second type of bone marrow
depression caused by chloramphenicol?

275 Anti-inflammatory agents strongly associated
with the development of aplastic anaemia include phenylbutazone, oxyphenbutazone and
amidopyrine. These are dangerous drugs and
the last two should no longer be used, whereas
the first should be used only when there is a
strong specific clinical indication. It is not
possible to predict which patients will develop
aplastic anaemia when treated with these drugs.
   Other agents predictably cause bone marrow
depression in a dose-related manner. What are
these?

276 The first essential step in the management of
aplastic anaemia is to identify and remove any
causative agents such as drugs or chemicals.
Transfusions are usually not required unless the
haemoglobin falls below 7 g/100 ml. Infections
should be treated rapidly and vigorously with
IV antibiotics, and platelet transfusions may
be required for haemorrhage.
   What general measures should be used to
avoid infection and haemorrhage in patients
with aplastic anaemia?

277 Androgens may benefit a considerable proportion of children with aplastic anaemia but are
much less helpful in adults. However, an
empirical trial of an androgenic agent such as
oxymethalone 2.5 mg/kg/day is indicated in
most cases for a period of 4–6 months.
   What is the treatment of choice in severe
aplastic anaemia?

Iron deficiency anaemia

278 Management of iron deficiency anaemia starts
with identification and treatment of the cause.
This is commonly due to menstrual or gastrointestinal blood loss. Once this has been done
the best way to treat the iron deficiency itself
is by giving ferrous iron salts orally. Ferrous
sulphate or gluconate preparations are suitable
and a dosage of 200–250 mg/day of elemental
iron should be the goal if the patient can
tolerate this.
   What are the side effects of oral iron
therapy?

279 The vast majority of patients with iron deficiency should be treated with, and will respond
to, oral iron therapy. However, parenteral iron
is available for those who genuinely cannot
tolerate the oral form or who cannot absorb
oral iron, i.e. some patients with malabsorption,
ulcerative colitis, Crohn's disease and intestinal
shunts.
   What adverse effects may follow parenteral
iron therapy?

280 The absorption of oral iron is enhanced by
ascorbic acid and alcohol but inhibited by tea,
tetracyclines and antacids.
   In which situations may it be hazardous to
administer iron and folic acid respectively?

Megaloblastic anaemia

281 The minimum daily requirement of folic acid is
50–100 µg/day. Pregnant women need about
400 µg/day. The therapeutic dose for treating
folic acid deficiency with megaloblastic anaemia
is 1–5 mg/day and 4–6 weeks' treatment is
usually enough to correct anaemia and replace
body stores.
   Which patients require long-term maintenance therapy with folic acid?

282 Vitamin B_{12} must be given to patients who
have had either a total gastrectomy or resection
of the terminal ileum.
   What is the difference between hydroxocobalamin and cyanocobalamin and why may
potassium supplements be needed during the

initial treatment of pernicious anaemia with B_{12}?

283 Hydroxocobalamin is the drug of choice in treating pernicious anaemia. A dose of 1000 μg IM should be given every day for 2 weeks in order to replenish body stores. Thereafter, 1000 μg IM 2-monthly is required for life.

How soon can a response be expected following initiation of treatment in a patient with pernicious anaemia?

Thrombocytopenia

284 Severe spontaneous bleeding is unusual with thrombocytopenia unless the platelet count falls below 20,000/mm^3 or some additional coagulation disorder is present. In general, therefore, platelet transfusions should be reserved for patients with thrombocytopenia who have severe haemorrhage or who require surgery.

What is the average half-life of transfused platelets? How many units should be given to an average adult with bleeding due to a platelet count below 10,000/mm^3?

285 Chronic ITP should be treated initially with high doses of prednisone (about 100 mg/day for an adult). This should be continued until the platelet count rises to 100,000/mm^3 or more and then it is gradually tapered.

What are the indications for splenectomy in ITP?

286 Important causes of drug-induced agranulo-cytosis include amidopyrine, antithyroid drugs, dapsone and to a lesser extent indomethacin, phenylbutazone and co-trimoxazole. This effect is mediated via damage to neutrophils or their precursors and is idiosyncratic rather than dose-related. Although the white cell count returns to normal on stopping the offending drug in the majority of cases, there is a very real risk of death from sepsis and vigorous antibiotic therapy may be required if infection develops.

Which drugs are important causes of thrombocytopenia?

287 Thrombotic thrombocytopenic purpura (TTP)

is a rare disease which usually occurs in young women. It is similar in some respects to the haemolytic uraemic syndrome (HUS) which, however, usually occurs in infants. Features of TTP include haemolysis, thrombocytopenia, fever, neurological disturbance and renal failure. It may follow an infection or the use of oral contraceptives.

How can TTP be treated?

Haemolysis

288 The anaemia of hereditary spherocytosis can be cured by splenectomy. However, because of the risk of pneumococcal infections and septicaemia this operation should be deferred at least until after the age of 5 years.

Should all affected children have splenectomy? What precautions can be taken to prevent infections following splenectomy?

289 Glucose-6-phosphate dehydrogenase deficiency is a sex-linked defect in which the principal feature is haemolysis produced by oxidant drugs such as sulphonamides, nitrofurantoin, primaquine phosphate, chloramphenicol and some vitamin K preparations. This disorder is common in blacks, orientals and individuals from the Mediterranean and Middle East.

What else apart from oxidant drugs may precipitate haemolysis in individuals with G6PD deficiency?

290 Warm autoantibody haemolytic anaemia is associated with a positive Coombs' test and the presence of IgG antibodies on the surface of the patient's red cells. It may be idiopathic or secondary to disorders such as SLE, lymphoma or ovarian teratoma.

Which drugs may cause autoimmune haemolytic anaemia and by what mechanism do they cause it?

291 Steroids are the treatment of choice for idiopathic autoimmune haemolytic anaemia. About 15% of cases fail to respond to steroids and should be considered for splenectomy.

What is the place of blood transfusions in autoimmune haemolytic anaemia?

292 Cold agglutinin haemolytic anaemia is associated with a positive Coombs test and an IgM anti-body. Precipitating causes include *Mycoplasma pneumoniae* and infectious mononucleosis.

How should cold agglutinin haemolysis be managed?

293 Paroxysmal nocturnal haemoglobinuria is a rare form of intravascular haemolysis in which red cells are excessively sensitive to complement-induced lysis. Diagnosis is confirmed by finding a positive Ham test. Complications include thromboses, infarctions and haemolytic or aplastic crises.

How should this disorder be managed?

294 Haemolytic reactions to blood transfusions can produce a variety of symptoms of which the most characteristic is loin pain. When such a reaction occurs or is suspected a number of investigations must be carried out. These include rechecking the donor blood matching, Coombs test, and urine and serum free haemoglobin levels on the recipient.

How should such a reaction be managed?

295 Methaemoglobinaemia occurs when more than 1% of an individual's haemoglobin contains iron which has been oxidized to the ferric form which cannot carry oxygen. Exposure to oxidizing agents such as aniline dyes and nitrates produces anaemia and cyanosis.

How should acute methaemoglobinaemia be treated?

Coagulation disorders

296 Vitamin K deficiency is a common cause of an acquired coagulation disorder leading to excessive bleeding. Causes of vitamin K deficiency include liver disease, malabsorption and alteration of normal gut flora. The main laboratory finding is a prolonged prothrombin time but levels of factors II, VII, IX, and X are also low.

How is bleeding due to vitamin K deficiency managed?

297 Haemophilia A (factor VIII deficiency) is treated by infusion of factor VIII concentrates. Minor cuts and bruises require no specific

therapy. More serious haematomas or haemar-
throses necessitate raising the patient's factor
VIII level to about 50% of normal and repeat-
ing the dose of factor VIII concentrate required
to achieve this 12-hourly for up to 4 days.

What level of factor VIII should be aimed
for in life-threatening haemorrhage or prior to
surgery or when haematomas occur in dangerous areas such as the neck?

298 Adverse effects from therapy are a problem in
the management of haemophilia. The use of
cryoprecipitate containing factor VIII may be
associated with the development of hepatitis
B and hepatitis non-A and non-B. Allergic
reactions including bronchospasm and rashes
are also a problem. Haemophiliacs are also at
increased risk of developing the acquired
immunodeficiency syndrome (AIDS).

Why should aspirin never be given to a
haemophiliac?

299 Von Willebrand's disease is an autosomal dominant disorder in which there is decreased factor
VIII activity and impaired ristocetin platelet
aggregation. Bleeding is usually less serious than
in haemophilia.

How should Von Willebrand's disease be
managed?

300 Disseminated intravascular coagulopathy (DIC)
is an acquired bleeding disorder due to intravascular activation of the coagulation system
with consumption of platelets and clotting
factors. Laboratory findings include thrombocytopenia, prolonged prothrombin time (PT),
partial thromboplastin time (PTT) and thrombin
clotting time, the latter indicating hypofibrino-
genaemia, and elevated levels of fibrin degradation products (FDPs).

How should DIC be managed?

Haemoglobinopathies

301 General management of a child with sickle cell
anaemia includes adequate diet and avoidance
of cold, dehydration and excessive physical stress.
Infections should be prevented as far as possible
by a full immunization programme and when infection does occur it should be treated promptly.

What regular medication should be given to sicklers? What specific travel advice should they be given?

302 Painful (infarctive) crises in sickle cell anaemia are due to entangled sickle cells lodging in small vessels causing vascular obstruction. This may occur at any site, although bones and spleen are commonly affected.

How should a painful sickle cell crisis be managed?

303 A child with severe β thalassaemia major may be treated by a high-transfusion programme which aims to keep the haemoglobin level at 9–14 g/100 ml in order to promote normal growth and development and reduce the risk of infections, and retard the development of hepatosplenomegaly. However, repeated transfusions eventually lead to iron overload with myocardial, hepatic and endocrine damage.

How may iron overload be prevented or minimized in this situation?

304 It is very difficult to get significant quantities of iron out of the body, the only ways being venesection and the chelating agent desferrioxamine. 500 cc of blood contains 200–250 mg of iron, whereas 1 g of desferrioxamine chelates up to 85 mg of iron. When anaemia is present, venesection is not acceptable.

What is the dose of desferrixoamine by subcutaneous infusion?

Myeloproliferative disorders

305 The initial treatment of polycythaemia rubra vera (PRV) is repeated venesection of 500 ml of blood two or three times a week in order to lower the PCV to below 0.5. Patients who have an elevated platelet count, or those with ischaemic features, should receive 500 ml of high molecular weight dextran twice weekly in order to expand plasma volume and prevent thrombosis. Once PCV is under control myelosuppressive therapy should be given.

What form may this take?

306 Treatment of myelofibrosis is generally unsatis-

factory. Folate deficiency is common due to rapid turnover, and folic acid supplements in a dose of 5 mg/day may be useful. Androgens may benefit an occasional patient and steroids may help if haemolysis or thrombocytopenia are a problem. Pyridoxine may help anaemia occasionally.

What is the place of myelosuppressive therapy and splenectomy in the treatment of myelofibrosis?

Malignant Disease

Chemotherapeutic agents

307 Alkylating agents appear to act by inhibiting DNA cross-linkage in tumour cells. The group includes cyclophosphamide, mustine, melphalan, chlorambucil, busulphan and procarbazine. Members of the group are useful in the treatment of a wide variety of tumours including leukaemias and lymphomas, myelomas and breast and ovarian cancer. One serious side effect of cyclophosphamide is haemorrhagic cystitis and even eventual bladder cancer.

What is the mechanism of this cystitis and how may it be prevented?

308 Vinca alkaloids such as vincristine and vinblastine act by precipitating microtubules and depressing protein synthesis, thus arresting dividing cells in metaphase. Vincristine is useful in treating acute lymphocytic leukaemia, lymphomas, and small cell undifferentiated lung tumours.

What are the main toxic effects of this group of drugs?

309 *Cis*-platinum is a potent antitumour agent which is useful in treating testicular, ovarian, bladder and some head and neck tumours.

What precautions must be observed when using this agent?

Radiotherapy

310 Radiation therapy is the initial treatment of choice for a variety of malignant disease includ-

ing the earlier stages of Hodgkin's disease, seminomas, some cases of cancer of the cervix, some bladder tumours and many head and neck tumours. Impressive cure rates have been achieved using radiotherapy in some of these diseases.

What is the place of radiotherapy in the palliation of malignant disease?

Leukaemia

311 Remission can be achieved in 90% of children with acute lymphoblastic leukaemia by a 4–6-week course of chemotherapy which includes vincristine, prednisolone, L-asparaginase and daunorubicin.

How may the development of meningeal leukaemia be prevented?

312 Various chemotherapeutic regimes are available for remission induction in acute myeloblastic leukaemia. One such regime includes daunorubicin, cytosine arabinoside and thioguanine.

What results can be expected from such therapy?

313 Chronic myeloid leukaemia is a biphasic disease with an initial chronic phase during which the patient can usually be maintained in fairly good health, followed by a subsequent acute or transformed phase during which there is rapid deterioration.

What is the usual therapy for the chronic phase?

314 The course of chronic lymphatic leukaemia is quite variable, and asymptomatic cases who are free of complications do not require specific therapy but should be observed.

What treatment is available for patients with constitutional symptoms or symptomatic lymphadenopathy?

Hodgkin's disease

315 The most important factor to consider when deciding initial management of Hodgkin's disease is staging. Additional factors are the

histological type of tumour, the age of the patient and the volume of disease present.

What type of patients would be expected to do well with radiotherapy alone?

316 Treatment for Hodgkin's disease stages, IIB, III and IV should include combination chemotherapy with a regime such as MOPP (mustine, vincristine, procarbazine and prednisolone). Other alkylating agents such as cyclophosphamide or chlorambucil may be substituted for mustine and may be less toxic.

What serious long-term complication may follow such regimes?

Gynaecological malignancy

317 Two to five per cent of all cases of gestational trophoblastic neoplasm lead to choriocarcinoma and 10% to invasive mole (chorioadenoma destruens). Thus careful follow-up of all cases from whom a hydatidiform mole is removed is essential. Serum β-human chorionic gonadotrophin (β-hCG) must be checked at weekly intervals until levels become undetectable, and monthly thereafter for a year. Other follow-up measures include regular gynaecological examinations and chest X-rays.

How should one treat choriocarcinoma?

318 Approximately 6% of all ovarian tumours are found to be malignant and primary ovarian carcinoma accounts for about 1 in 5 of all gynaecological cancers.

What general guidelines apply to management of ovarian malignancy?

Testicular tumours

319 Testicular cancer is frequently curable but early diagnosis is essential and any testicular swelling must be regarded as malignant until proven otherwise. Seminoma is very radiosensitive and is treated by excision of the affected testis followed by radiation to paraaortic lymph nodes if they are involved.

How does the treatment of malignant teratoma differ from this? How should patients with testicular cancer be followed up after therapy?

Breast cancer

320 A commonly used approach to the treatment of breast cancer includes mastectomy and removal of axillary lymph nodes.

The place of adjuvant chemotherapy remains under discussion, but can you suggest a reasonable approach?

Cancer of the prostate

321 Cancer of the prostate is very common in older men and treatment depends on the stage of the disease. If the cancer is confined to the prostate, radical prostatectomy or external irradiation may be used.

What additional treatment is recommended for patients with lymph node or visceral metastases?

Multiple myeloma

322 Treatment of multiple myeloma includes intermittent 4-day courses of melphalan and high-dose steroids.

How should this therapy be monitored?

Bone marrow transplantation

323 Bone marrow transplantation is a very useful form of therapy in leukaemia. However it is necessary to have an HLA identical sibling as a donor and the recipient must be in haematological remission.

How is the procedure carried out?

324 One of the main problems following bone marrow transplantation is the development of graft versus host disease. Features of this include enteritis, hepatitis and exfoliative dermatitis.

Which drug is most useful in controlling graft versus host disease?

Immunosuppression and infection

325 Fever developing in severely immunocompromised patients such as those on chemotherapy for malignant disease must be presumed to be due to infection unless proven otherwise. For patients with severe granulocytopenia ($<500/mm^3$) cultures from relevant sites (blood, urine, throat and any other suspicious area) must be obtained immediately and antibiotics must be administered at once without awaiting culture results.

What is a reasonable antibiotic regime to use while awaiting culture results?

Malignant pleural effusion

326 Malignant pleural effusions may be due to lymphatic obstruction or direct tumour invasion of the pleura.

How may they be treated?

Rheumatological Disorders

Septic arthritis

327 A 22 year old marine commando develops a painful left elbow. Arthrocentesis reveals purulent synovial fluid with many Gram-negative cocci on microscopy. He is allergic to penicillin.

What antibiotic would you recommend while awaiting culture results?

328 A 60 year old man with a 30-year history of insulin-dependent diabetes mellitus develops a painful swollen left knee. Arthrocentesis reveals cloudy white fluid, with a synovial fluid white cell count of $90,000/mm^3$ of which 90% are polymorphonuclear leucocytes. Microscopy of this fluid also reveals Gram-positive cocci.

How would you manage him?

329 A 58 year old woman has been on a low dose of steroids for rheumatoid arthritis for 6 years. She presents to you with fever and an acutely painful left knee with a joint effusion, and a

leucocytosis of $20,000/mm^3$ in the peripheral blood.

What test will you do next and what therapy will you consider?

Rheumatoid arthritis

330   Gold therapy is indicated in patients with severe rheumatoid arthritis whose symptoms cannot be controlled by NSAIDs alone and in whom penicillamine has been discontinued due to side effects.

What precautions are necessary with gold therapy?

331   You are working as a medical intern in a district hospital. You are assisting a rheumatologist with his outpatient clinic, when he is called away urgently, leaving you alone. One patient remains to be seen, a 35 year old female teacher with severe rheumatoid arthritis. She has been on penicillamine for 6 months and has now developed proteinuria.

How will you manage her?

332   Steroids are potent anti-inflammatory drugs and they can produce a major improvement in symptoms in rheumatoid arthritis.

What are the indications for systemic steroid therapy in rheumatoid arthritis?

333   Patients with severe rheumatoid arthritis who cannot tolerate gold or penicillamine therapy should be considered for cytotoxic drug therapy with azathioprine or cyclophosphamide.

What precautions are necessary when using azathioprine?

Osteoarthritis

334   Osteoarthritis is commonly treated with NSAIDs. However, other measues are important in managing this disease.

What are these?

335   The advantages of total hip joint replacement are excellent pain relief, maintenance of mobility and rapid postoperative recovery.

What are the disadvantages and complications of this operation?

Seronegative arthropathies

336 Salicylate therapy is usually ineffective in controlling the pain of ankylosing spondylitis. Indomethacin is the most effective drug with an acceptable level of side effects.

What other measures are important in the management of ankylosing spondylitis?

337 One month after a visit to Bangkok, a 24 year old businessman develops urethritis, conjunctivitis and arthritis. You make a diagnosis of Reiter's syndrome. The patient has a history of asthma since childhood, and also has had a nasal polypectomy on two occasions during the past 5 years.

Should you treat his arthritis with aspirin?

Connective tissue disorders

338 Mild SLE should be treated conservatively. Joint pains, fever and inflammation of serosal membranes often respond to NSAIDs.

What is the place of hydroxychloroquine in the therapy of SLE?

339 Therapy with systemic steroids in SLE should be reserved for cases with complications such as severe glomerulonephritis, CNS or myocardial involvement, and severe haemolysis or thrombocytopenia.

What is 'pulse' therapy?

340 Drug-induced lupus differs from the naturally occurring variety in that whereas the ANA test is positive in both, there are no antibodies to double-stranded DNA in the drug-induced variety.

Which two drugs are most commonly implicated in drug-induced SLE and which individuals are especially prone to this reaction?

341 Systemic sclerosis is a collagen disease in which response to therapy, in particular with steroids, is very poor. However, a certain GIT complication does improve with medication.

What is this?

342 Polyarteritis nodosa (PAN) is a necrotizing form of vasculitis which involves medium-sized

arteries. Mortality is high unless treatment is commenced early.

What forms of therapy are useful in PAN?

343 A 75 year old man complains of pain and stiffness in the shoulders, buttocks and back. His symptoms are worse in the morning and on examination there is considerable tenderness of muscles in these areas. In addition, he complains of constant headache, blurring and transient loss of vision in the left eye. His ESR is 100 mm/hour.

How will you manage him?

Gout and pseudogout

344 Indications for lifelong allopurinol therapy for hyperuricaemia include recurrent attacks of gout, tophaceous gout, uric acid nephropathy and uric acid nephrolithiasis.

What precautions are necessary when using allopurinol?

345 A 55 year old businessman has had three acute attacks of gout over a period of 6 months. He has therefore been commenced on allopurinol therapy. Two weeks later, however, he develops fever and a diffuse exfoliative dermatitis.

What will you do?

346 The following drugs cause hyperuricaemia by decreasing renal excretion of uric acid: diuretics, low doses of salicylates 1–2 g/day), pyrazinamide and ethambutol.

How would you manage an acute attack of gout in a patient on diuretics?

347 A 60 year old farmer has had several attacks of acute arthritis involving knees and wrists. Calcification is visible in the joint space on X-ray of his knees. Examination of synovial fluid from the left knee under a polarized light microscope reveals pleomorphic weakly positively birefringent crystals.

Is he likely to benefit from (a) allopurinol and (b) colchicine?

Soft tissue disease

348 A 60 year old carpenter complains of a painful
stiff shoulder. Examination reveals a painful
movement arc on abduction between 70° and
110°. All rheumatological investigations are
normal and you make a diagnosis of supra-
spinatus tendonitis.
   How will you manage him?

Non-steroidal anti-inflammatory drugs

349 Propionic acid derivatives such as ibuprofen and
naproxen are probably the best NSAIDs to start
with in treating arthritis. This is because this
group of drugs has the lowest incidence of side
effects.
   What are the benefits and side effects of the
cyclic acetic preparation indomethacin?

350 A 50 year old housewife has been on therapy
with propranolol and bendrofluazide for essential hypertension. Her blood pressure had
been well controlled on this regime but a week
after starting indomethacin for an osteoarthritic
knee, her blood pressure is 200/120.
   Could the rise in blood pressure be related to
the addition of indomethacin?

Intra-articular steroids

351 Intra-articular steroid injections are contraindicated in patients in whom there is any possibility of septic arthritis or who have evidence of
skin infection or sepsis elsewhere.
   How long does the benefit of intra-articular
steroids last?

Neurological Disorders

Headaches and migraine

352 Tension headache is the commonest form of
headache. Occasional episodes respond to simple analgesics but frequent or daily headaches
should be treated with regular small doses of a
tranquillizer, such as diazepam 2 mg three times
daily.

What else should be done for the patient?

353 The analgesic effect of aspirin and paracetamol is increased both by the use of dissolved preparations and by simultaneous administration of metoclopramide which stimulates gastric emptying. This combination of drugs is often effective in the early stages of a migraine headache. Once a migraine headache is established however, the most effective relief is provided by ergotamine.

What is the usual dose and what dangers attend excessive ergotamine intake?

354 Drugs or diet can be successful in preventing migraine attacks. Propranolol, clonidine in low doses and methysergide are useful prophylactics, although methysergide is liable to cause retroperitoneal fibrosis.

Which foods are commonly implicated in migraine and should be tested by exclusion from the diet?

355 Cluster headaches, also called migrainous neuralgia, tend to occur during the night and oral therapy taken at the time of attack is seldom very effective. Ergotamine can prevent the headaches if given parenterally or rectally before the headache begins, i.e. when the patient goes to bed.

What is the dose of ergotamine, either by injection or by suppository?

356 Headaches in older people may be due to temporal arteritis. Prompt initiation of corticosteroid therapy is important since this disease is a cause of blindness.

In which other neurological conditions are corticosteroids of undisputed value?

Analgesia

357 Morphine and pethidine are the most commonly used strong analgesics. Both drugs can be given by IV or IM injection and morphine has been used intrathecally for postoperative pain relief.

What common side effect is shared by both morphine and pethidine and how may it be overcome?

358　Following head injury or subarachnoid haemor-
　　rhage, analgesia may be required. The most
　　important observation in the clinical assessment
　　of patients with these conditions is the level of
　　consciousness, and potent analgesics all tend
　　to cause some drowsiness and sedation.
　　　　Which injectable analgesic is least likely to
　　cause sedation, but always leads to constipa-
　　tion?

359　Causalgia, or 'phantom limb' pain, often
　　responds to transcutaneous nerve stimulation
　　(neuroelectric therapy).
　　　　Which other treatment may be successful?

Insomnia

360　In the treatment of insomnia the benzodiaze-
　　pines have replaced barbiturates as the drugs
　　of choice. Insomnia may consist of difficulty
　　getting to sleep, in which case a rapid but
　　short-acting drug is indicated, or early waken-
　　ing, when a drug with a more prolonged dur-
　　ation of action is required.
　　　　What is the duration of action of flurazepam,
　　temazepam and nitrazepam?

Epilepsy

361　In the treatment of epilepsy the goal should be
　　to prevent seizures with one drug alone. Mix-
　　tures or combinations of drugs produce complex
　　interactions, many of which may decrease the
　　effectiveness of the drugs given.
　　　　What is the therapeutic range of phenytoin
　　concentration in the plasma?

362　In adults with grand mal epilepsy the most
　　commonly used drug is phenytoin. Which two
　　newer drugs each offer good alternative single-
　　drug therapy?

363　In the treatment of petit mal epilepsy, which
　　usually occurs in children, it is desirable to
　　avoid mental dulling and impairment of learn-
　　ing ability. Ethosuximide is the usual drug of
　　choice, but its main side effect unfortunately
　　is drowsiness.
　　　　What drug can be used in its place?

364 Carbamazepine is an anticonvulsant effective in grand mal, temporal lobe and Jacksonian epilepsy. A typical adult starting dose is 100 mg twice daily but it induces its own metabolism and the dose should be gradually increased in the first 4 weeks. It also induces the metabolism of other drugs including warfarin.

In which other neurological condition is carbamazepine used?

365 Chlormethiazole is a sedative and anticonvulsant with a half-life under 1 hour. By continuous IV infusion it is an easily controlled therapy for delirium tremens, and it can also be used for status epilepticus if the first-choice drugs have failed.

What drugs should be used initially in the treatment of status epilepticus?

Cerebrovascular disease

366 Transient ischaemic attacks due to platelet emboli may be prevented by anti-platelet agents although it is not certain that this alters the incidence of strokes. Apart from aspirin, dipyridamole is used.

What is a typical adult dose and what are the main side effects?

367 In cerebral artery thrombosis, cerebral vein thrombosis and venous sinus thrombosis the use of anticoagulants carries a danger of haemorrhage from an area of infarction.

In which cerebral event is anticoagulation usually strongly indicated?

368 In the rehabilitation of patients suffering from a stroke, physical and occupational therapy and sometimes speech therapy are of prime importance in maintaining fitness and the patient's interest in life, and in helping him to make up for the disability.

In the early stages of a hemiplegia what form of physical therapy is essential?

Parkinsonism

369 The three main features of Parkinsonism are rigidity, akinesia and tremor. Levodopa usually

improves akinesia and rigidity whereas the anticholinergic drugs benzhexol, orphenadrine and benztropine may reduce tremor. These drugs should not be used for drug-induced extrapyramidal reactions.

What is the treatment for these reactions other than withdrawal of the causative drug?

370   In idiopathic Parkinsonism the effectiveness of levodopa is increased by the addition of a dopa-decarboxylase inhibitor. This allows more of the administered dopamine to escape peripheral degradation and enter the brain.

What are the dose-limiting side effects of levodopa?

371   Bromocriptine stimulates dopamine receptors in the brain. It is sometimes effective in patients with idiopathic Parkinsonism who cannot tolerate the side effects of levodopa.

In which other conditions is bromocriptine of therapeutic value?

Cerebral oedema

372   Dexamethasone is one of the most potent anti-inflammatory corticosteroids. Approximately 3 mg of dexamethasone is equivalent to 20 mg of prednisone. Its most important indication is in the reduction of cerebral oedema associated with cerebral contusion, cerebral tumour or benign intracranial hypertension.

What is the usual adult dose and what may the patient notice immediately after IV injection?

Myasthenia gravis

373   The weakness of myasthenia gravis is improved by prolonging the action of acetylcholine with anticholinesterase drugs. Neostigmine and pyridostigmine are the drugs commonly used.

How are they taken and what is the usual adult dose?

Essential tremor

374   Benign familial or essential tremor is marked by

a complete absence of other neurological findings. It improves with alcohol consumption.
Which drug brings at least some improvement in most cases?

Narcolepsy

375 Dexamphetamine is a drug of addiction and its
use in adults should be confined to the treatment of narcolepsy. Too much of the drug
causes unwanted wakefulness.
What recommendations would you give to
a narcoleptic patient for whom you are prescribing dexamphetamine?

Infectious and Tropical Diseases

Meningitis and encephalitis

376 Ninety per cent of bacterial meningitis is due to
infection with the meningococcus (a Gram-
negative intracellular diplococcus) or the pneumococcus (a Gram-positive diplococcus).
What is the treatment of choice for these
two forms of meningitis?

377 *Haemophilus influenzae* is a Gram-negative
bacillus which may cause bacterial meningitis,
usually in children under the age of 6 years.
The treatment of choice for this form of meningitis is chloramphenicol 50–100 mg/kg/day
for 5 days followed by 30 mg/kg/day for a
further 5 days.
What are the major pathogens in neonatal
meningitis and what is the treatment of choice?

378 Tuberculous meningitis is usually fatal unless
treated effectively. The two anti-TB drugs
which pass most effectively into the CSF are
isoniazid and pyrazinamide, and these should
be given along with rifampicin and streptomycin for 2–4 months followed by rifampicin
and isoniazid for 8 months. Pyridoxine 10 mg/
day should also be given to prevent isoniazid-
induced peripheral neuropathy.
What is the place of steroids in the treatment
of TB meningitis?

379 The most dangerous form of herpes simplex infection is herpes simplex encephalitis. It produces a haemorrhagic encephalitis mainly involving the temporal lobes.

What drugs are available to treat herpes simplex encephalitis?

Gastrointestinal infections

380 In giardiasis and amoebiasis, metronidazole is the treatment of choice. This drug is also indicated in anaerobic infections.

In which intestinal infection is vancomycin the first-choice antibiotic?

381 Antibiotic therapy is contraindicated in uncomplicated salmonella gastroenteritis.

Why is this?

382 The major requirement for effective therapy of cholera is early and rapid rehydration. Mild cases who are not vomiting respond well to an oral electrolyte solution containing sodium chloride, sodium bicarbonate, potassium chloride and glucose. More seriously ill cases require large volumes of IV fluid through a large-bore cannula. A cut-down may be necessary for this.

What is the value of antiobiotics in the management of cholera?

383 Shock, altered consciousness and severe toxaemia indicate a poor outlook in patients with typhoid fever. Very high doses of IV dexamethasone (e.g. a stat dose of 3 mg/kg followed by eight doses of 1 mg/kg every 6 hours) for the first 2 days of treatment, in addition to chloramphenicol, appear to cause a marked improvement in the survival of such patients, and thus are strongly indicated.

How should one manage the carrier states of typhoid fever?

384 The treatment of choice for the majority of cases of typhoid fever is chloramphenicol 500 mg every 4 hours until fever disappears, followed by 500 mg 6 hourly for a total of 14 days. However, chloramphenicol-resistant strains of *Salmonella typhi* have recently appeared, especially in Latin America, and in

addition chloramphenicol occasionally causes fatal aplastic anaemia.

What alternative antibiotics are available for treating typhoid fever?

385 A 30 year old businessman develops diarrhoea 5 days after returning to Britain from a business trip in India. The diarrhoea is not bloodstained but is associated with abdominal cramps and nausea. He decides to seek your opinion when he finds that diarrhoea persists, despite over-the-counter remedies from the chemist. Microscopic examination of his stool reveals oval double-walled cysts 8×12 μm in size, containing two to four nuclei and rudimentary flagellae.

How would you manage him?

Viral infections

386 A 21 year old female medical student comes to you with a 2-week history of sore throat and fever. Two days before presentation, she took some ampicillin. This was rapidly followed by development of a widespread maculopapular erythematous rash. On examination, she has a marked pharyngeal exudate, slight splenomegaly and a few palatal petechiae. She is not anaemic.

What is the main test indicated in this situation and how would you manage her if the result is positive?

387 Yellow fever vaccine is a live attenuated vaccine, and it confers protection for 10 years.

What are the contraindications to this vaccine?

Bacterial infections

388 Diphtheria can be very successfully prevented by active immunization with diphtheria toxoid. However, the disease can be extremely dangerous in the non-immunized and may lead to respiratory obstruction, circulatory failure, myocarditis, paralysis and severe toxaemia.

How should diphtheria be managed?

389 Good nursing care is of vital importance in the management of severe pertussis, especially in

infants. The child should be turned head-down during cough spasms in order to prevent aspiration. Feeding should be done following spasms because vomiting tends to occur at the end of each spasm.

What is the place of antibiotics, antitussives and anticonvulsants in the treatment of pertussis?

390 Important measures in treating tetanus include treatment of the precipitating wound by debridement and high doses of penicillin.

What is the place of human tetanus immunoglobulin (HTIG) in the treatment of tetanus?

391 Patients with leprosy may be divided into two groups according to the number of bacilli present. In patients with multibacillary disease (lepromatous or borderline lepromatous leprosy), leprosy bacilli can readily be found in skin and ear lobes. In contrast, bacilli are hard to find in patients with paucibacillary disease (tuberculoid and borderline tuberculoid leprosy).

How does drug therapy of these two forms of leprosy differ?

392 The commonest haematogenous organism causing acute osteomyelitis is *Staphylococcus aureus*. However, *Streptococcus pyogenes* and Gram-negative organisms may also be responsible. Thus it is reasonable to commence therapy following the taking of cultures with an antistaphylococcal agent such as clindamycin or flucloxacillin, plus an aminoglycoside if Gram-negative infection is suspected.

By which route should treatment be given, and for how long?

393 Pneumoccocal disease carries a significant morbidity and mortality and prevention is desirable.

Vaccination with a polyvalent pneumococcal vaccine has been recommended for patients with chronic cardiac, respiratory and hepatic disease. In which two groups of patients is vaccination particularly indicated?

Fungal infections

394   In the immunocompromised host lung infections are frequently due to opportunistic
organisms such as *Pneumocystis carinii*,
Aspergillus fumigatus, *Candida albicans* and
Nocardia asteroides.
    To which antibiotics are these separate
organisms sensitive?

395   Amphotericin B is the drug of choice for treating many systemic mycoses including histo-
plasmosis, coccidiomycosis and cryptococcosis.
As it is not absorbed from the GIT it must be
given parenterally.
    What are the main adverse effects of
amphtotericin B?

Rickettsial infections

396   A 21 year old zoology student develops fever
and headache a few days after returning to
Europe following an elective period of field
studies in Indonesia. There is an eschar over-
lying a painless ulcer on his left ankle and the
inguinal glands on the left are swollen and
tender. There is a maculopapular truncal rash.
The Weil–Felix reaction with OXK is positive.
    The patient is allergic to tetracycline. How
will you treat him?

397   Both tetracycline and chloramphenicol are
effective in treating Rocky Mountain spotted
fever, but tetracycline is the treatment of
choice due to its less serious side effects.
    What important factors should be borne
in mind when treating this disease?

Protozoal infections

398   Toxoplasmosis usually causes a mild self-
limiting illness when it occurs in previously
healthy adults and antimicrobial treatment
is not indicated. However, infection in pregnant
women or immunocompromised patients is
more serious.
    How should these be managed?

399   The treatment of choice for amoebic dysentery

consists of metronidazole 400 mg tid for 5 days
plus diloxanide furoate 500 mg tid for 10 days.
Metronidazole has an amoebicidal effect both
in the tissues and in the lumen of the gut,
wheareas diloxanide furoate acts only on
amoebae in the gut lumen.

What management would you suggest for an
individual who is asymptomatic but who is
passing amoebic cysts in the stool?

400 A 30 year old photographer, recently returned
from a 6-month tour of South East Asia, complains of fever and pain in the right hypochond-
rium and right shoulder. His liver is enlarged
and tender, and investigation reveals a raised
ESR and polymorphonuclear leucocytosis.
Chest X-ray shows a raised right hemidiaphragm.

What is the likely diagnosis? How will you
confirm it? What is the treatment?

401 The main feature of *Leishmania tropica* infection is the development of indurated skin
ulcers. One infection produces immunity for
life but may be followed by ugly scarring.

How can the disease be treated?

402 The drug of choice for treating visceral
leishmaniasis is one of the pentavalent antimony preparations such as sodium stibglucon-
ate or *N*-methylglucamine antimonate.

What features are of value in monitoring the
response to this therapy?

403 Treatment of African sleeping sickness is not
very satisfactory. Suramin is effective in the
early stages of both East and West African
trypanosomiasis, and pentamidine is useful in
the therapy of early cases of *Trypanosoma
brucei gambiense* infection. However, neither
drug is effective against neurological complications.

How can the neurological stage of African
sleeping sickness be treated?

Malaria

404 General measures, such as use of mosquito net-
ting and wearing long sleeves and trousers, help
reduce the risk of contracting malaria. However, such measures by no means eliminate the

danger altogether, and any non-immune individual should take prophylactic tablets when travelling through or residing in a malaria zone.

How would you advise a girl who is 2 months pregnant and who intends to travel to West Africa for a month, but who is worried about possible damage to her baby by anti-malarial tablets?

405   A 30 year old engineer develops fever, headache, rigors and vomiting 2 weeks after returning to Europe from Papua New Guinea. Examination of a thin blood smear shows 15% of his red blood cells contain malaria parasites and some gametocytes are visible.

How would you manage him?

406   A 21 year old student who visisted southern India 18 months ago develops fever and splenomegaly. A thin blood smear reveals malaria parasites within red blood cells, some of which are enlarged and contain Schuffners dots.

What is the likely form of malaria? What is the treatment?

407   Proguanil and pyrimethamine are prophylactic antimalarial drugs which have very low toxicity in the doses normally used. The former is taken on a daily basis, the latter weekly. Unfortunately, many strains of *Plasmodium falciparium* which are resistant to chloroquine also display resistance to these antifolate preparations.

What advice would you give to a European missionary who has spent the last 5 years working in West Africa and who has taken 300 mg of chloroquine base weekly during this period?

Worm infestations

408   A 19 year old Cameroonian boy complains of haematuria. Microscopic examination of his urine reveals eggs of 135 μm in length with a sharp terminal spine.

How would you treat him?

409   Oxamniquine is a relatively non-toxic anti-schistosomal drug which is highly effective against *Schistosoma mansoni.*

What is the value of this preparation in the overall control of schistosomiasis?

410 The best drug for treating lymphatic filariasis is diethylcarbamazine citrate (DEC–C). It kills both microfilariae and adult worms and may be used for treating symptomatic individuals and for mass treatment. However it has a serious drawback when used for mass treatment of asymptomatic infected people.
What is this?

411 Diethylcarbamazine kills microfilariae but not adult worms when used in onchocerciasis (African river blindness).
What is the Mazzotti reaction and how may its severity be reduced?

412 A 40 year old Australian male complains of an itchy red serpiginous skin eruption which appears to migrate slowly in the skin. He first noticed this 20 years ago during a period of military service in New Guinea, but it has been more troublesome over the past few months. Examination of a stool specimen reveals mobile rhabditiform larvae.
How would you treat him? What medications are strongly contraindicated?

413 Hydatid disease carries a risk of rupture of cysts leading to anaphylaxis or dissemination of larvae. Surgical enucleation of the cysts is the treatment of choice.
In situations where the disease is far advanced or the patient is unfit for surgery, what can be done for him?

414 You are asked to see a 5 year old African boy who recently arrived in Europe from Nigeria. He has a history of abdominal discomfort and occasional diarrhoea. His haemoglobin is 8 g% with a microcytic hypochromic blood picture and eosinophilia of 10%. Examination of a stool specimen reveals large numbers of oval eggs 60 μm in length with a smooth outer capsule.
What does this clinical picture suggest? How would you manage him?

415 A heavy infection with *Ascaris lumbricoides* in a child may produce malabsorption and limit growth.

How would you diagnose and treat infection with *Ascaris?*

416 A mother brings a 6 year old child to you because he has been restless at night. On questioning you discover that the restlessness is due to severe perianal itching and excoriation. You suspect threadworm infection.

How would you confirm this diagnosis and what would be your management?

417 Niclosamide is regarded as the drug of choice for tapeworm (cestode) infections. It is usual to give 2 g orally, taken on an empty stomach.

What theoretical risk applies to use of this drug in *Taenia solium* infections?

Zoonoses

418 Leptospirosis is a zoonotic disease due to infection with one of the spirochaetes of the genus *Leptospira.* Diagnosis may be confirmed by blood culture which may be positive in the first week, or by urine culture which may be positive in the third week of illness. A rising titre of antibodies in the serum after the second week confirms this diagnosis.

How relevant are these investigations to therapy?

419 Anthrax is a zoonotic disease due to the anaerobic Gram-positive spore-forming bacterium *Bacillus anthracis.* It is an occupational hazard for farmers and those processing carcases and hides. There are two forms: firstly the 'malignant pustule' and secondly 'wool sorter's disease', which is a haemorrhagic pneumonia due to inhalation of anthrax spores.

How should anthrax be managed?

420 Tetracycline in large doses, e.g. 500 mg 4–6 hourly for 3 weeks, is probably the best treatment available for acute brucellosis. Subacute brucellosis (i.e. where the illness lasts more than a month), may respond to a combination of tetracycline and streptomycin.

What can be done for chronic brucellosis?

421 Rabies is virtually always fatal. A very small

number of cases are known to have recovered but these were treated in high-technology intensive-care units. Unfortunately, most cases of rabies occur in areas where such facilities are non-existent.

How should rabies be managed in such circumstances?

422 Thorough wound cleaning is one of the most important first aid measures in rabies prevention.

Can you outline the procedure for post-exposure prophylaxis against rabies in a patient not previously immunized against rabies who is bitten by a rabid animal?

Sexually transmitted diseases

423 The treatment of genital herpes is not very satisfactory. Idoxuridine, while benefiting labial herpes, is not effective in genital herpes.

What is the value of acyclovir in treating genital herpes?

424 Gonorrhoea may be treated by procaine penicillin 4.8 megaunitis IM plus probenecid 1 g orally 30 min before the injection. Alternatively, amoxycillin 3 g orally plus probenecid 1 g orally is also effective. While this therpy may seem simple and straightforward, certain other measures are essential in addition.

What are these?

425 Penicillin is the treatment of choice for all stages of syphilis. For primary and secondary syphilis, 600,000 units of procaine penicillin should be given IM for 10 days. The same regime applies to early latent syphilis (under 2 years) but late latent syphilis requires the same dosage for 15 days and neurosyphilis and cardiovascular syphilis require 20 days therapy. Patients with latent syphilis who have difficulty attending for daily injections may be treated with benzathine penicillin 2.4 megaunits IM once weekly for 3 weeks but this regime is inadequate for neurosyphilis and cardiovascular syphilis.

How may patients with penicillin allergy be treated? What is the Jarisch–Herxheimer reaction?

426   In some areas non-specific urethritis (NSU) is a commoner cause of urethritis in men than gonorrhoea. Many cases of NSU appear to be due to infection with *Chlamydia trachomatis* (TRIC agent).

      What therapy should be used for NSU and what is the prognosis?

Drug reactions and interactions

427   A 20 year old youth with epilepsy has been seizure-free on phenytoin sodium 100 mg tid. However 1 day following commencement of sulphonamide therapy for a urinary infection, he suddenly becomes ataxic.

      Can you explain why?

428   Most fatal anaphylactic reactions to penicillin occur in individuals without a previous history of penicillin allergy. Many patients with a history of allergy have later been successfully treated with penicillin without any evidence of allergy.

      How then can one avoid major reactions to penicillin and how should one approach the management of a patient with the history 'allergic to penicillin'?

429   A 70 year old man is known to have poly-myalgia rheumatica. This has been well con-trolled on 5 mg of prednisolone daily. He then develops tuberculosis and is started on anti-tuberculous chemotherapy, including rifampicin. His polymyalgia rheumatica flares up 3 weeks later.

      Why?

Skin Disorders

430   The treatment of pruritus is generally unsatis-factory but topical therapy is useful in the presence of inflammatory skin disease such as eczema.

      What is the value of systemic medication for pruritus?

431   Topical steroids are the most effective treat-ment for atopic eczema, but they carry the risk of systemic side effects. Thus the weakest

possible preparation which is effective should be used.

How would you manage (a) a 1 year old baby with extensive eczema on the limbs and (b) a 40 year old man with severe eczema confined to the hands?

432 A 19 year old female student comes to you with severe acne on her face and trunk. Over the past 2 years she has taken several courses of antibiotics, including tetracycline and erythromycin, and she has used numerous topical preparations without significant benefit. She is now very depressed and anxious because of her condition.

What other measures are available for treating severe acne?

433 A 30 year old woman complains of disfiguring psoriatic plaques on the face.

Should one prescribe dithranol or topical steroids in this situation?

434 Certain vitamin A derivatives are useful in psoriasis. Etretinate appears to be especially useful in pustular psoriasis of palms and soles. It may be used alone or combined with PUVA (psoralens and ultraviolet light).

In which individuals is this drug especially contraindicated?

435 Psoralens such as 8-methoxypsoralen, when given orally, combine with pyrimidine bases in skin exposed to ultraviolet light to form cross-linkages and inhibit DNA synthesis. This is the mechanism of action of PUVA therapy in psoriasis.

What precautions are necessary when using PUVA therapy?

436 Dermatitis herpetiformis causes severe itching. The response to dapsone is usually rapid and dramatic. However side effects of dapsone are serious and they include haemolysis, agranulocytosis, rashes, peripheral neuropathy and GIT upset.

What additional measure is indicated in dermatitis herpetiformis?

437 Staphylococcal impetigo may be treated effectively by debridement of crusts and cleansing

of the skin combined with a topical antibiotic such as bacitracin. Systemic antibiotics are rarely necessary.

How should streptococcal impetigo be treated?

438 Scabies should be treated by applying 1% gamma-benzene hexachloride or 0.25% benzyl benzoate to the entire body surface below the neck on two occasions 24 hours apart.

What additional measure is essential?

439 Hereditary angioedema is an autosomal dominant disorder due to C1 esterase inhibitor deficiency. The most dangerous complication is laryngeal oedema which may be fatal.

How can this disorder be treated?

440 A wide range of cutaneous drug reactions may occur. These include exanthematic reactions to drugs such as antibiotics, sulphonamides and gold, and bullous reactions which may be induced by agents such as barbiturates, iodides and nalidixic acid.

How should a patient with a cutaneous drug reaction be managed?

441 Among the important iatrogenic causes of alopecia are cytotoxic agents, heparin and coumarin, propylthiouracil, oral contraceptives, sodium valproate, beta blockers and levodopa.

Which agents may cause hypertrichosis?

Eye Disorders

442 It is important to avoid giving topical cortico-steroids to patients with corneal ulceration as this can lead to blindness in cases due to herpetic keratitis.

How should herpes simplex keratitis be managed?

443 Trachoma is a very common cause of blindness in the developing world. It is due to infection of the conjunctiva with *Chlamydia trachomatis*. This gradually leads to scarring, entropion and trichiasis. Control of trachoma includes public health measures such as provision of an adequate clean water supply and hygienic living conditions.

How should the infection be treated in the individual patient?

444 Infection with the dog nematode *Toxocara canis* may produce a retinal mass similar to a retinoblastoma and may lead to blindness. There is usually an associated eosinophilia.
     How should this infection be treated?

445 Anterior uveitis is usually a fairly benign condition which responds well to mydriatics and steroid eye drops. Posterior uveitis is more serious and all cases should be carefully invest- igated for evidence of serious underlying disease. If a specific cause such as an infection is identified this should be treated appropriate- ly.
     How should one manage progressive, recur- rent or severe uveitis or uveitis associated with impairment of vision?

446 Chronic simple (primary open-angle) glaucoma causes gradual painless loss of peripheral vision. Management may be medical or surgical (filtration surgery). Medical preparations in- clude the following eye drop solutions: miotics such as pilocarpine, sympathomimetics such as adrenaline, and beta blockers such as timolol which reduces production of aqueous humour.
     How should an acute attack of closed-angle glaucoma be treated?

ENT Disorders

447 Extrinsic allergic rhinitis is a hypersensitivity disorder due to external allergens. Symptoms include sneezing, nasal obstruction and rhinorrhoea.
     How can this condition be managed?

448 Acute tonsillitis is commonly due to viral in- fection with agents such as adenoviruses. Some cases are due to infection with haemolytic streptococci.
     How should acute tonsillitis be managed?

449 Features of acute sinusitis include a purulent nasal discharge with nasal obstruction, facial pain and tenderness and puffiness of the cheek.

How should acute sinusitis be managed?

450 Otitis externa is an extremely painful infection of the skin of the external auditory canal. It is common in tropical climates and following swimming.

How should otitis externa be managed?

451 Acute otitis media mainly occurs in children and is usually secondary to upper respiratory tract infection. Many cases resolve without specific therapy but it is advisable to give antibiotic treatment early in order to achieve a rapid resolution and avoid complications.

Which antibiotics should be used in the treatment of acute otitis media?

Nutritional Disorders

Vitamins

452 A major physiological role of vitamin A is the control of cell differentiation. There is some evidence that beta carotene, a precursor of vitamin A, may protect against certain forms of cancer, particularly lung cancer.

However it is important that people should avoid excessive consumption of vitamin A in an attempt to prevent cancer. Why is this?

453 Some health-conscious individuals may consume massive doses of vitamin C because of claims that it may prevent the common cold or prevent cancer. The evidence for these effects is extremely slender.

How may this form of self-medication be harmful?

454 Certain people who are at risk of developing osteomalacia should be considered for vitamin D prophylaxis. These include the elderly, the mentally handicapped in institutions, post-gastrectomy patients and epileptics on long-term treatment with phenytoin or phenobarbitone.

What are the toxic effects of large doses of vitamin D?

455 The only clinical manifestation of vitamin K

deficiency is haemorrhage. Confirmation of
deficiency is made by noting the response
to vitamin K administration.

What side effects may occur with vitamin K?

Obesity

456 Semistarvation diets of 800 kilocalories per day,
especially when combined with an exercise
programme, have a high success rate in enabling
obese individuals to lose weight.

In what conditions are such severely restricted diets contraindicated?

457 Fenfluramine is an amphetamine derivative
used in treating obesity. It has an anorectic
effect but it is also a sedative.

How effective is fenfluramine therapy in
obesity?

458 Appetite suppressants are often requested by
patients but, if used at all, they should be
considered only as a temporary measure. Di-
ethylpropion is related to amphetamine but
seldom causes tremor or restlessness although
addiction and psychosis have been described.

Fenfluramine, although also related to
amphetamine, has mild sedative properties.
What features occur in sudden withdrawal of
large doses of fenfluramine?

Hyperalimentation

459 Provision of nutritional support for a patient
who cannot swallow or tolerate oral feeding
can be successfully achieved by giving enteral
feeds by gravity infusion through a fine-bore
polyurethane nasogastric feeding tube.
Although these newer tubes appear free of complications such as oesophageal erosions and
strictures, which occurred with older large-bore
tubes, modern enteral nutrition is not free of
complications.

What are these?

460 One of the serious complications which occurs
with parenteral nutrition is catheter-related
sepsis.

What precautions can reduce the risk of this
occurring?

461 Fat emulsions are a useful energy source in patients on parenteral nutrition. However, the proportion of a patient's total caloric intake from this source should not exceed 60%. The remainder should come from glucose and protein solutions.

In which conditions are parenteral fat emulsions contraindicated?

462 Patients with sepsis or serious injuries who are on parenteral nutrition may develop severe hyperglycaemia and hyperosmolar dehydration. This is related to high levels of circulating insulin antagonists including adrenal steroids, growth hormone, glucagon and catecholamines.

How may this problem be controlled?

Poisoning and Snakebite

Poisoning/toxicology

463 Gastric lavage should only be performed on an unconscious patient after the insertion of a cuffed endotracheal tube. It is worth doing for up to 12 hours after ingestion of salicylates, antidepressants and anticholinergic substances, and for up to 4 hours in the case of other substances.

How should adsorbents be used in cases of poisoning?

464 Naloxone is a specific antidote for narcotic overdosage. It is effective against all opiates such as morphine and heroin but it is also useful in overdosage of non-narcotics such as dextropropoxyphene and pentazocine.

What precautions should be taken when treating a patient with naloxone?

465 A 2 year old boy is brought to hospital after swallowing up to 20 of his mother's iron tablets. You carry out gastric lavage, after which a solution of desferrioxamine in saline is left in the stomach.

What additional measures are indicated?

466 Forced alkaline diuresis is effective in treating

poisoning due to drugs which are excreted unchanged in the urine, such as salicylates and phenobarbitone. It is of no value for drugs which are metabolized to inactive metabolites.

What rate of urine flow, and what urine pH, should one aim for with forced alkaline diuresis?

467 An 18 year old university student presents 5 hours after taking a paracetamol overdose. His plasma paracetamol taken on arrival at the hospital casualty department is 300 mg/ml.

What treatment is indicated and how does it work?

468 In cases of digoxin overdosage, measurement of plasma digoxin 6 hours following ingestion provides a good indication of prognosis. Virtually any cardiac arrhthmia can occur in digoxin intoxication.

Which antiarrhythmic agent is most useful in management of digitalis-induced ventricular arrhythmias?

469 When a patient on digoxin shows an arrhythmia consisting of two or more abnormalities, e.g. atrial tachycardia with AV block, or if the ventricular rhythm becomes regular in atrial fibrillation, digoxin intoxication should be suspected.

How may digoxin overdosage be treated?

470 Continuous ECG monitoring of patients who have ingested an overdose of tricyclic preparations is essential because of the risk of fatal arrhythmias.

How should such arrhythmias be managed?

471 A 35 year old accountant is brought to hospital by his wife. He complains of vomiting, diarrhoea, abdominal colic, dyspnoea and sweating. His pulse rate is 40/min and his pupils are constricted. On questioning his wife you discover that he had been spraying fruit trees in his garden with parathion 2 hours previously, and due to warm weather he had been stripped to the waist.

How will you manage him?

472 Charcoal haemoperfusion is an effective new technique for treatment of poisoning. Blood

is pumped through an albumin-coated charcoal filter which absorbs large amounts of toxins. This method should be considered in cases with severe poisoning or those with underlying hepatic or renal impairment.

With which substances is charcoal haemoperfusion of definite benefit and what are its side effects?

473 Antifreeze contains ethylene glycol or methanol or both. These are metabolized in the body to the toxic metabolites oxalic acid and formic acid respectively.

A 25 year old mechanic ingests 300 ml of antifreeze. What therapy, apart from general measures, is indicated?

Snakebite

474 Vipers are snakes such as the European adder which have long erectile fangs. The venom of these snakes is vasculotoxic.

What are the indications for using antivenom in patients with viper bite?

475 Elapids are snakes such as cobras, mambas and kraits which have short unmoving fangs. The venom of these snakes has neurotoxic effects (paralysis, dysphagia, respiratory paralysis) or necrotizing effects leading to necrosis of skin in the area of the bite.

What is the value of arterial tourniquets, or incision or freezing of the bitten skin?

476 Antivenom is only indicated in cases of snakebite with evidence of systemic poisoning, but signs of this must be carefully sought, and once they appear antivenom must be given without delay.

What precautions are necessary in the use of antivenom?

Disorders due to physical agents

477 The underlying disorder in the malignant hyperthermia syndrome seems to be an increase in the concentration of calcium ions in the sarco-

plasmic reticulum of skeletal muscle. It is usually precipitated by halogenated inhalational anaesthetic agents and by the muscle relaxant succinyl choline.

How should this syndrome be managed?

478 A 10 year old boy is brought to a hospital emergency room following near-drowning in a polluted river.

How would you manage him?

479 A 30 year old nuclear power station worker suffers heavy contamination with radioactive liquid following an accident.

What immediate measures would you suggest and what treatment may he require?

480 A 30 year old climber has been rescued following a night spent on a mountainside in a blizzard. His feet appear to be frostbitten.

How would you manage him?

481 Slow rewarming at room temperature is indicated in cases of mild hypothermia (core temperature above 32° C). More severe cases may benefit from hot humidified oxygen.

What IV fluids would you recommend for a patient with hypothermia and what is the place of antibiotics in this situation?

Pregnancy and Lactation

482 Teratogenicity can be hard to prove, and when uncertainty prevails, the reluctance to take medications displayed by many women is to be praised. (This intelligent non-compliance also complicates the problem of proving teratogenicity.)

Which analgesic, tranquillizer and antibiotic appear to be least likely to harm the fetus?

483 It is often assumed that the passage of maternal drugs into breast milk does not matter because maternal illness usually causes an interruption in breast-feeding. Use of a breast-pump to maintain lactation, however, may make this assumption incorrect.

Which drugs are of particular concern?

484 During pregnancy, a diabetic woman's glucose
levels need to be closely monitored and insulin
doses adjusted to her individual requirements.
The requisite obsessional care in this respect
carries a slight risk of hypoglycaemia but
maternal hypoglycaemia has not been shown
to be harmful to the fetus whereas maternal
ketoacidosis frequently causes intrauterine
death.

How would you control the blood glucose
during labour?

485 Although oedema is often a prominent feature
of severe pre-eclampsia, diuretics are contraindicated.

Why is this and what it the one exception to
this general rule?

486 Severe chronic renal failure is a cause of infertility but pregnancy in milder cases is not uncommon. The increased obstetric morbidity
found in chronic renal failure appears to be related to the degree of accompanying hypertension rather than to the renal impairment.

In what way does the treatment of hypertension in pregnancy differ if renal failure is
present?

487 Fear of teratogenic effects has traditionally
limited antihypertensive therapy in pregnancy
to the long-established drugs alphamethyldopa
and hydralazine.

What has been the theoretical objection to
using beta blockers in pregnancy?

488 Most epileptic mothers taking phenytoin de-
liver normal infants although there is a slightly
increased risk of fetal abnormality. In general
the fetal risk from uncontrolled maternal
epilepsy is considered greater than the fetal
risk from phenytoin. Plasma phenytoin levels
tend to fall during pregnancy but an increase
in phenytoin dosage is seldom necessary.

Why is this?

489 Anticoagulation in pregnancy is a difficult
problem. Both heparin and warfarin carry
some risk for the fetus.

In a woman with a mitral valve prosthesis
who is already taking warfarin what is the
ideal management of her anticoagulation

during pregnancy, delivery and the puerperium?

490 The majority of abnormal fetuses caused by warfarin exposure during the first trimester are aborted spontaneously. This means that the fetal damage most commonly seen after warfarin therapy in pregnancy is haemorrhage.

Why is the fetus susceptible to warfarin damage?

491 Sickle cell disease and other severe haemolytic anaemias carry a raised obstetric morbidity. Present thinking favours a policy of hyper-transfusion during pregnancy.

What is the rationale for this?

Psychiatric Disorders

Anxiety and depression

492 Acute anxiety states usually respond to discussion of the anxiety and an anxiolytic drug such as oral diazepam.

Which additional drug is useful when somatic manifestations of anxiety, such as tachycardia or sweating, become troublesome?

493 Depression is most often treated either with tricyclic or with tetracyclic compounds.

How do these two groups of drugs differ with respect to drug interactions and speed of onset of therapeutic effect?

494 Monoamine oxidase inhibitors are effective antidepressants but may be the cause of fatal drug interactions.

Name a drug interaction involving an over-the-counter medicine.

495 When treating hypertension in a patient with depression it is better to avoid drugs which can cause mood changes and other features of depression. Such drugs include reserpine, alpha-methyldopa and clonidine.

Which antihypertensive drugs are safe in this regard?

496 Patients taking tricyclic antidepressants often

experience anticholinergic side effects, namely dryness of the mouth, blurring of vision, constipation and, especially in older men, urinary retention.

What is the most common neurological side effect of phenothiazine drugs and how can it be prevented?

Psychotic disorders

497 The sudden presentation of acute psychosis may necessitate treatment before psychiatric help is available. The drugs of choice are chlorpromazine and haloperidol.

In a young adult man what would the starting dose of each drug be?

498 Chlorpromazine and other phenothiazines all share a large number of side effects, of which extrapyramidal reactions and jaundice are the most frequently encountered.

What effect does chlorpromazine have on the peripheral vasculature?

Alcoholism

499 Delirium tremens not uncommonly occurs when a heavy drinker is unexpectedly admitted to hospital. It is marked by tremulousness and tactile and visual hallucinations.

Which drugs are best for controlling alcohol withdrawal symptoms?

500 Patients with Wernicke's encephalopathy require urgent admission to hospital for treatment. This consists of parenteral thiamine 50–100 mg daily.

How long should thiamine be continued? How may doctors precipitate Wernicke's encephalopathy?

Cardiovascular Disorders

Angina pectoris

1   In states of severe volume overload, left
    ventricular dilatation or raised LVEDP, the
    left ventricle may be maintaining output by
    virtue of adrenergic stimulation via the beta
    receptors. Blockade of these receptors will
    lead to worsening heart failure. In cases of
    doubt, beta blockers should initially be admin-
    istered in small doses with close monitoring.

2   A headache confirms the drug's potency and if
    no headache occurs the dose may be inadequate.
    Severe headaches may be managed by reduction
    of the dose. Oral paracetamol is often helpful.
    Sometimes increasing the frequency of doses,
    e.g. to every 3 hours, lessens the headaches by
    causing a more sustained and stable vaso-
    dilatation.

3   Nitrites and nitrates oxidize haemoglobin to
    methaemoglobin (but significant methaemo-
    globinaemia is uncommon).

4   Heart rate may increase while heart size decreases
    due to reduction in venous return. There is a re-
    duction in myocardial oxygen demand and this
    explains the effectiveness of these drugs although
    coronary artery dilatation can also occur.

5   Empirically, starting with a dose of 10 mg three
    times daily. Theoretically the drug can also re-
    duce perfusion of ischaemic myocardium,
    either by lowering diastolic blood pressure or by
    dilating healthy coronary arteries more than
    narrowed arteries and causing coronary steal.

In each patient the most effective dose should be established by trial.

Myocardial infarction

6   Bed-rest in semi-sitting position, oxygen, IV 5% dextrose in the minimum quantity necessary to keep a vein open, and a liquid or soft low sodium diet as tolerated. A stool softener given daily will help to avoid prolonged straining at stool which may be a cause of arrhythmias.

7   IM administration takes 20–30 min to begin to be effective and with the reduced tissue perfusion that accompanies hypotension absorption will be delayed. A smaller dose of the drug (5–10 mg) should be administered IV to give an immediate and predictable effect. IM injections also cause a slight elevation of creatine kinase which may cause diagnostic confusion. A further caveat is that ischaemic pain may be more effectively relieved by a pure vasodilator such as IV nitroglycerine.

8   Five per cent dextrose in water is the solution least likely to embarrass a weakened heart since it contains no sodium and this advantage more than offsets the incidence of drip-site phlebitis seen with dextrose solutions. The minimum flow needed to keep a vein open is 5–10 cc per hour. This should be controlled by a pump so that the patient is protected from accidental administration of excess fluid.

9   Dopamine should be commenced at 1 or 2 μg/kg/min and increased at 5 min intervals until a rise in blood pressure is obtained. A large dose would be 20 μg/kg/min. The dose is regulated according to the response.

10 Increased levels of circulating free fatty acids have been shown to cause arrhythmias. Insulin reduces these levels. In addition there is experimental evidence that insulin and dextrose therapy can limit infarct size.

11 Increased fluids should be given to augment right ventricular output. Some advocate giving albumin to further increase circulating volume and right ventricular filling.

12   By attention to correct procedure. Pulmonary
      infarction can occur if the balloon is left in-
      flated by mistake or if the tip of the catheter
      becomes permanently wedged. A daily chest
      X-ray should be done to check catheter
      position.
          A long thrombus may develop in the cathe-
      ter lumen if regular flushing is neglected. Sub-
      sequent expulsion of the thrombus may cause
      clinically significant embolism. Regular flush-
      ing with or without heparinization of the
      flushing solution should prevent this.

13   The development of left axis deviation in this
      setting indicates left anterior hemiblock, which
      is in·addition to the existing RBBB. In anti-
      cipation of possible complete heart block a
      temporary pacing wire should be inserted.

14   Coronary artery flow is maximal during dia-
      stole and depends on diastolic aortic pres-
      sure (as well as the duration of diastole). In-
      flation of the balloon in the aorta increases
      proximal aortic pressure and coronary artery
      perfusion pressure.

15   It seems likely that sternal compression pro-
      duces a cardiac output (up to 30% of normal)
      by raising intrathoracic pressure and it may be
      logical therefore to splint the diaphragm by
      pressing on the abdomen. When ventricular
      fibrillation occurs during cardiac catheteriz-
      ation, continuous shallow coughing may main-
      tain consciousness.

16   Give 5000 units SC every 8 hours. Monitoring
      of clotting parameters is unnecessary.

17   This question is still disputed. It would seem
      reasonable for a patient without complications
      (not even sinus tachycardia) to remain 2
      weeks, while the development of complications
      should mean a stay of up to 4 weeks or longer.

18   The two main high-risk groups are those with
      critical narrowing of the left main coronary
      artery and those with triple vessel disease.

19   Beta blockers, and anti-platelet drugs (aspirin,
      sulphinpyrazone, dipyridamole).

20   (a) Exercise should be increased slowly but steadily, increments being defined in terms of the patient's own environment; e.g. if there is a flight of stairs at home, the number of journeys up and down should be specified.

      (b) By the time a patient leaves hospital, he or she should be fit enough for modest sexual activity.

      (c) Return to work after 1–3 months' convalescence is reasonable, the time depending on the severity of the infarction.

21   The increased anaesthetic risk to a patient with a myocardial infarction continues to diminish for 6 months after the infarction, so surgery and general anaesthesia should be delayed at least 6 months if possible.

Congestive cardiac failure

22   In the presence of sinus rhythm there is no reliable way to judge the dose of digoxin (in contrast to observation of the ventricular rate in atrial fibrillation). Plasma digoxin levels are a guide to the likelihood of toxicity being present ($> 2\mu g/l$) but they do not take account of individual susceptibility. The positive inotropic effect may not be achieved due to overcautious underdosage, or it may be overshadowed by morbidity due to digoxin toxicity.

23   A transient rise in blood pressure may occur within the first few minutes, followed by venous dilatation and reduction of venous return to the heart after 10–15 minutes.

24   Approximately 6–8 hours. The therapeutic effect of digoxin appears to be related to the tissue levels rather than the high plasma levels that immediately follow oral or IV administration.

25   Quinidine alters digoxin pharmacokinetics by reducing renal excretion and reducing volume of distribution, resulting in raised serum digoxin levels.

26   In the presence of renal impairment, hypoalbuminaemia (digoxin is one-third protein-bound) and during anaesthesia due to inter-

action with anaesthetic agents, particularly muscle relaxants.

27   All of these side effects can be caused by both drugs. Spironolactone is probably more likely to cause gynaecomastia while digoxin only causes headaches and gastrointestinal symptoms when tissue levels are excessive.

28   Captopril. This drug blocks the conversion of angiotensin I to the active angiotensin II. The first few doses should be given cautiously. Maximal effect is achieved with 150 mg a day in divided doses and higher doses do not carry any additional benefit.

29   Potassium-sparing diuretics, namely spironolactone, amiloride and triamterene, and vasodilators, namely nitrites, hydralazine and prazosin.

30   A thiazide diuretic with a milder but longer duration of action may be acceptable and equally effective. The diuretic effect of chlorothiazide is spread over 6–12 hours while that of chlorthalidone may last 24–48 hours.

31   Thiazide diuretics (chemically related to sulphonamides) impair glucose tolerance, reduce net renal excretion of uric acid and can cause light-sensitive dermatitis.

32   Vasodilators (principally prazosin, hydralazine and nitrites) reduce after-load (and pre-load in the case of nitrites). Reducing the work of a failing left ventricle improves cardiac output and renal perfusion. The stimulus to aldosterone production thus declines and diuresis ensues.

33   Venesection. Rapid removal of 300–500 cc of blood may relieve pulmonary oedema but has the disadvantage of reducing the oxygen-carrying capacity of the blood. In renal failure patients with no response to diuretics, dialysis is indicated, but may take longer to arrange than an immediate venesection.

34   A vasodilator such as hydralazine or prazosin. These drugs are both antihypertensives and effective after-load reducing agents. Beta

blockers are contraindicated because of her left ventricular failure and, to a lesser extent, because of her insulin-dependent diabetes.

35   When sodium losses due to diuretics exceed sodium intake over a prolonged period of time, sodium depletion may occur. This reduces renal perfusion and reduces the effectiveness of diuretic therapy. The patient may then be unable to excrete his customary water load and oedema worsens. In this situation sodium administration (as oral sodium chloride) may restore the effect of diuretics.

Cardiac arrhythmias

36   Propranolol in small doses, or verapamil.

37   Quinidine, which prolongs the refractory period of atrial muscle. Disopyramide also has this effect.

38   IV verapamil (1 mg/min up to 10 mg).

39   Surgical removal or ablation of the accessory pathway.

40   Atropine, by IV injection. An average dose would be 0.8 mg.

41   Add 1 mg of isoprenaline to 250 ml of 5% dextrose in water.

42   The initial bolus of lignocaine is 50–100 mg for an adult. Although opinions vary on the rate of infusion, the short half-life of lignocaine makes it logical to establish adequate blood levels with 4 mg/min for 30 min, then reducing to 2 mg/min. Subsequent adjustments up to a maximum of 4 mg/min are made according to the response.

43   Yes, in company with all other drugs which depress myocardial function.

44   Mexiletine has a half-life of 16–18 hours, while that of lignocaine is only 1–2 hours. Common side effects include nausea and tremor.

45   Disopyramide has some anticholinergic activity

which can precipitate urinary retention in the presence of prostatic hypertrophy. This is approximately as troublesome a problem as the SLE syndrome induced by procainamide.

46   The half-life of procainamide is short (3 hours) and effective therapy means a dose every 3 hours. It is not practicable for patients to take medication at night, and this is one of the reasons for this drug being used less often. It can also cause a reversible SLE syndrome.

47   Phenytoin (250 mg IV over 3–5 min) or bretylium (250–500 mg IV as necessary up to a maximum of 1.5 g in any 24 h).

48   Amiodarone may be effective. The high incidence of side effects (pneumonitis, resistant ventricular tachycardia, sinus arrest, sinus bradycardia, ataxia, nausea and potentiation of digoxin and warfarin) make it suitable only for arrhythmias resistant to other anti-arrhythmic agents.

49   Lignocaine, disopyramide or phenytoin are usually effective. Beta blockers are also effective but are considered by some to be contraindicated because of the risk of increasing the AV block which may already be present due to digoxin.

50   There is no ideal treatment for idioventricular rhythms. Although they are worrying as possible preludes to more serious arrhythmias. treatment is not free of the risk of precipitating a more harmful arrhythmia. Atropine, by blocking the vagal effect on the SA and AV nodes, may speed up the atrial rate and allow the atria to recapture the ventricles. This may also be achieved by slowing the ventricular rate with lignocaine. Anterior infarction is a more worrying setting for idioventricular rhythms than inferior infarction.

51   The patient should be informed and be lying flat with an IV line patent. Sedation is induced with IV diazepam. Atropine and lignocaine should be drawn up ready to give in the event of bradycardia or ventricular extrasystoles respectively.

52   A temporary pacemaker should be inserted so
      that the heart can be driven in the event of
      complete heart block.

53   Beta blockers (e.g. propranolol), verapamil,
      procainamide and occasionally amiodarone.

Hypertension

54   The blood pressure should be checked on at
      least another two occasions, since initial read-
      ings can be misleadingly high. His lifestyle
      and eating habits should be ascertained with
      a view to helping him to lose weight and, if
      sedentary, take more exercise. In addition
      simple screening tests should be done to look
      for the commoner causes of secondary hyper-
      tension and to check for the presence of any
      other cardiovascular risk factors.

55   In the first days of therapy, depletion of
      circulating volume reduces blood pressure but
      the renin–angiotensin–aldosterone system is
      stimulated and this then opposes the purely
      diuretic effect. Subsequently maintenance of
      an antihypertensive effect may be due in part
      to a vasodilator action. This weakens, however,
      with long-term therapy because of gradual
      potassium and magnesium depletion.

56   The potassium-sparing diuretics are more expen-
      sive than some (but not all) of the thiazides.
      They tend to have side effects which the
      patient is more likely to notice, e.g. nausea and
      dizziness, whereas thiazides are better
      tolerated.

57   It has been shown that the natriuretic hormones
      or agents, previously referred to as 'the third
      factor' can cause vascular smooth muscle con-
      traction as well as sodium excretion.
          In practice, dietary sodium restriction is of
      unpredictable benefit.

58   Logically blockade of beta receptors in blood
      vessels by leaving alpha receptors unopposed
      should lead to vasoconstriction. Although beta
      blockers can worsen Raynaud's phenomenon,
      peripheral vasoconstriction is seldom a problem.
      Renin production is reduced by beta blockade

but the most important action appears to be a central one on synapses in the vasomotor centre. The negative chronotropic effect on the heart may play a part in some patients.

59 Hypertension due to a phaeochromocytoma is the result of intensive alpha adrenoreceptor stimulation. Beta blockade will effectively augment this.

60 Hydralazine is a vasodilator. It reduces afterload on the left ventricle but in reducing systemic pressure it may provoke reflex tachycardia. Concurrent administration of a beta blocker, particularly propranolol, blocks the reflex tachycardia.

61 Spironolactone is an aldosterone antagonist and blocks the secondary aldosteronism provoked by the thiazide alone.

62 Captopril blocks angiotensin-converting enzyme, preventing the formation of angiotensin II.
   Captopril plus a diuretic is a logical and effective combination.

63 Alpha methyldopa needs to be taken three times a day to give 24 hour control of blood pressure. Sedation is a common side effect and hepatotoxicity and Coombs-positive haemolytic anaemia are uncommon but important side effects. The drug possesses no additional cardioprotective properties (in contrast to beta blockers or hydralazine) and it interferes with investigations for phaeochromocytoma. Depression can occur, especially in elderly patients.

64 The first dose of prazosin is 1 mg and it should be taken when the patient has got into bed. This is because the first dose can cause profound postural hypotension.
   Good compliance is important to avoid repeated first-dose side effects.

65 Purists decry combination preparations, arguing rightly that it is important to adjust the drugs separately to meet a patient's individual needs. In practice, however, the better compliance observed with a smaller number of tablets often outweighs the benefits of keeping the drugs separate.

66   Avoidance of abrupt cessation of therapy which
      may cause a hypertensive crisis. Such a crisis
      should be treated by alpha blockers. When
      clonidine therapy is being withdrawn the dose
      should be reduced gradually.

67   The doctor must show by his actions that he
      is convinced of the seriousness of the hyper-
      tension. It is all too easy for a doctor to wash
      his hands of a non-compliant patient but this
      may actually convey to the patient the im-
      pression that his blood pressure doesn't really
      matter. The doctor must persist with close
      follow-up, different combinations of drugs
      and a continuous effort to find a way to solve
      the patient's problem.

68   Biofeedback. This technique requires strong
      motivation and practice but some patients
      have undoubtedly used it successfully.

69   Correction of hypertension generally improves
      tissue perfusion due to autoregulatory
      mechanisms but this is not true of fixed arterial
      stenoses when lowering of blood pressure will
      reduce distal perfusion. The desirable level of
      blood pressure will need to be judged accord-
      ingly.

70   In an untreated patient it indicates autonomic
      neuropathy, adrenal insufficiency or acute loss
      of blood volume as in gastrointestinal bleeding.
          In a patient on antihypertensive therapy a
      postural fall in blood pressure is most com-
      monly due to excessive sodium loss from
      diuretics (since ganglion blockers are no longer
      in widespread use). In chronic renal failure also
      a postural fall is a sign of sodium depletion.

71   If a response occurs, it is seen within 15
      minutes.

72   Diazoxide needs to be given rapidly as a bolus.
      The usual dose is 300 mg but some prefer to
      give 150 mg first and follow with a second
      150 mg after 5 minutes if necessary. The dis-
      advantage of the drug is that one cannot titrate
      the dose with the effect. Excessive falls in pres-
      sure are encountered not infrequently, seriously
      compromising coronary, cerebral and renal
      perfusion.

73   In renal failure excretion of nitroprusside meta-
      bolites is impaired and accumulation will cause
      tinnitus, blurred vision and delirium. A meta-
      bolic acidosis on arterial blood gases is the
      earliest sign of cyanide toxicity.

74   The oral contraceptive, liquorice (often used
      as a laxative), carbenoxolone, corticosteroids
      and NSAIDs.

75   Percutaneous angioplasty. In this technique a
      catheter with a low-volume high-pressure
      balloon is advanced to the site of the stenosis
      and the balloon is inflated. Correction of a
      stenosis by any technique, however, does
      not always correct the hypertension.

Rheumatic carditis

76   Corticosteroids are virtually always effective,
      either alone or in addition to a reduced dose
      of salicylates.

Bacterial endocarditis

77   Ampicillin 1 g plus gentamicin 1.5 mg/kg IV
      30 minutes before the procedure, and repeated
      twice at 8-hourly intervals. The dose of genta-
      micin should be reduced in the presence of
      renal impairment.

78   For dental and ENT procedures, patients can
      receive a cephalosporin. If allergic to cephalo-
      sporins, vancomycin is recommended.
          For GUT and GIT and biliary tract pro-
      cedures, vancomycin and gentamicin should
      be used.

79   A combination of gentamicin 3–5 mg/kg/day
      (providing renal function is normal) plus
      penicillin G 20 megaunits/day for 6 weeks.

80   The mean inhibitory concentration for the
      synthetic pencillinase-resistant penicillins
      should be established. One of these may be
      suitable or, failing this, vancomycin and genta-
      micin are indicated.

Pericardial disease

81 Indomethacin, other NSAIDs or corticosteroids. Pericardial effusion with tamponade requires pericardiocentesis.

82 The three least dangerous sites for needle insertion are (i) 2 cm lateral to the apex beat in the 5th intercostal space; (ii) in the 5th or 6th intercostal space at the sternal border and directed medially; (iii) under the xiphisternum directing the point of the needle to the left shoulder and keeping it close to the wall of the chest.

Dissecting aneurysm

83 In acute aortic dissection the antihypertensive agent of choice is the ganglion blocker trimethapen. A solution containing 1 mg/ml in 5% dextrose should be used, with the patient in the sitting position.

Thromboembolic disease

84 There is no generally accepted regimen. An example would be 50 units per kg bodyweight loading dose followed by 12.5 units/kg/h by continuous infusion. Clotting time measurements should be performed frequently depending on the response.

85 Cholestyramine can bind warfarin in the gut and reduce absorption. Reduction of vitamin K levels (by broad-spectrum antibiotics) removes the antagonist to warfarin, increasing the anticoagulant effect. Displacement of warfarin from plasma protein-binding sites (by many drugs including aspirin) increases the availability of the drug. Competition for the same metabolic path in the liver (phenytoin, tolbutamide) increases the half-life. Cimetidine may potentiate the anticoagulant effect. Enzyme induction by barbiturates or alcohol will shorten warfarin half-life and oestrogen will also reduce warfarin effect by increasing clotting factors.

86   In the presence of active bleeding or within 2
      months of a cerebrovascular accident strepto-
      kinase must not be used. After an initial loading
      dose of 250,000 units (preceded by hydrocor-
      tisone) 100,000 units per hour is given for
      24–72 hours. Monitoring of clotting para-
      meters does not alter the dose.

Respiratory Disorders

Bacterial pneumonia

87   *Klebsiella pneumoniae*, unlike the pneumococ-
      cus, is not sensitive to penicillin. Antibiotic
      therapy should be changed to an aminoglycoside
      (e.g. gentamicin 80 mg IM or IV every 8 h) com-
      bined with a cephalosporin (e.g. cephazolin
      500 mg IM or IV every 6 h) and continued for
      10–14 days.

88   Delay in initiating treatment in Legionnaire's
      disease is associated with a high mortality. Thus
      erythromycin 0.5–1 g 6-hourly IV should be
      commenced when the diagnosis is suspected.
      This should be continued for 3 weeks. Assisted
      ventilation may be required also.

Pleurisy

89   The usual adult dose of indomethacin is 25–50
      mg three times daily. Dizziness, light-headed-
      ness and gastric intolerance are the most com-
      mon side effects.

Atypical pneumonia

90   *Mycoplasma pneumoniae*, *Chlamydia psittaci*
      and *Coxiella burneti* are all sensitive to
      tetracycline. Erythromycin is also effective
      against *Mycoplasma*.

Pulmonary tuberculosis

91   Serum uric acid levels rise due to a reduction in
      urinary excretion. Gout may be precipitated.

92 A transient abnormality of liver function tests is common at the initiation of therapy but this usually subsides without cessation of treatment. More serious disturbances of liver function can occur and nausea and vomiting may be trouble-some. Intermittent therapy, which should no longer be used, leads to the 'flu syndrome'.

Red discoloration of urine and tears is evidence only of drug ingestion. The half-life of concurrently administered warfarin, oestrogens (contraceptive pill) and steroids is reduced.

93 Isoniazid 300 mg/day for 6–12 months in adults. The dose in children is 5 mg/kg/day. Toxicity of this regime is rare except in alcoholics and individuals aged over 40.

Asthma

94 For outpatients using a pressurised inhaler, two puffs four times daily is the usual recommended dose. In hospital, the usual dose in a nebulizer is 2 ml of 0.5% solution. Side effects are tremor, tachycardia, dizziness and sometimes headache.

95 In pulmonary oedema due to severe mitral regurgitation. Salbutamol decreases peripheral resistance and this allows an increased pro-portion of left ventricular stroke volume to go into the aorta as opposed to the left atrium.

96 Metoprolol, acebutolol and atenolol are all cardioselective beta blockers.

97 There is a considerable individual variation but an average loading dose would be 6 mg/kg body-weight. This dose can be repeated 4-hourly or an equivalent amount can be diluted in IV fluids and given by constant infusion. Drug levels should be checked in the plasma.

98 The half-life of aminophylline is prolonged in the elderly and in the presence of liver disease. It is shortened in cigarette smokers. Half of the usual IV dose should be given if the patient has been taking one of the oral preparations as an outpatient.

99 A dose of 0.1 cc of 1 in 1000 adrenaline solu-

tion (equivalent to 180 μg) by subcutaneous injection.

100 Beclomethasone dipropionate and betamethasone valerate are topical steroids which can be inhaled as an aerosol from a pressurized 'puffer'. A typical starting dose would be one or two puffs three or four times daily. Oropharyngeal candidiasis can result but this usually responds to amphotericin B lozenges, one four times daily, or nystatin suspension, 1 ml four times daily.

101 In atopic asthma, in some cases of non-atopic asthma (in which the possible allergen is unknown) and in exercise-induced asthma. The starting dose is one capsule four times daily by inhalation through a special inhaler.

102 A usual starting dose is 4 mg three times daily but there is considerable individual variation in tolerance. The maximum therapeutic effect is not obtained until the patient has increased the dose to the point of drowsiness.

103 All possible measures to reduce the quantity of house dust should be carried out. These include daily or twice-daily cleaning with a vacuum cleaner, removal of carpets, regular cleaning of bedding, use of plastic-covered pillows and mattresses and adequate ventilation.

104 Sodium cromoglycate, salbutamol or verapamil. Corticosteroids are not effective.

105 The full treatment lasts 3–5 years with annual courses of injections timed to finish just before the anticipated onset of symptoms. Each course of injections consists of steadily increasing quantities of antigen(s).

Chronic bronchitis and emphysema

106 Amoxycillin 250–500 mg every 8 h, or cotrimoxazole, two tablets every 12 h or tetracycline 250–500 mg every 6 h. Ampicillin has the same spectrum of activity as amoxycillin but the latter is better absorbed and gives higher drug levels in the sputum.

107 Antibiotic-resistant strains of bacteria may develop. The diseased bronchi may become colonized by non-respiratory pathogens such as Gram-negative bacilli, posing a more difficult therapeutic problem.

108 A low dose of prednisone, 5–10 mg daily, is sufficient to give symptomatic improvement in conjunction with other therapy, i.e. chest physiotherapy, antibiotics, bronchodilators (where there is a reversible component to the airways obstruction) and avoidance of dust, smoke and other irritants.

109 Hydralazine can cause a reversible SLE syndrome with doses greater than 200 mg per day in men, but in women the safe limit is lower.
     There may be clinical and ECG evidence of reduced right ventricular strain, but the only certain way of judging the effectiveness of hydralazine is by measuring pulmonary artery pressure with a pulmonary artery flotation catheter (Swan–Ganz catheter).

110 The vaccine is prepared from viral cultures in chick embryos and contains some egg antigens.

111 Sheer will-power. Those who have given up smoking abruptly by will-power alone are least likely to resume.

Respiratory failure

112 Enough to raise the partial pressure of oxygen in arterial blood to approximately 7.3–8 kPa (55–60 mmHg). At this level tissue oxygenation and pulmonary vasoconstriction are both improved without depression of the respiratory centre. For each patient the dose of oxygen must be established empirically by checking arterial blood gas values frequently.

113 There is a sufficient margin of safety between relief of pain and respiratory depression to permit adequate use of these drugs. Linctus methadone may be particularly useful for suppressing a painful cough.

114 A clean suction catheter should be used for each insertion down the tube, thus avoiding

carriage of upper airway organisms to the trachea and bronchi.

115 Doxapram is given as an IV infusion up to 4 mg/min depending on the response.

116 Accidents can occur with ventilators, for example power failure or disconnected tubing. The paralysed or completely sedated patient with no spontaneous respiratory effort will immediately become anoxic. It is preferable to use the ventilator in an assist mode so that the patient's own breathing can continue. Intermittent mandatory ventilation (IMV) is one form of this.

117 Expiration, which is prolonged in asthma, must occupy more than 50% of the respiratory cycle but, within this restriction, inspiration must be as slow as possible to avoid unnecessarily high and dangerous inflation pressures.

118 In pregnancy, in the presence of high levels of progesterone, hyperventilation occurs. It is believed to be due to a direct action of the hormone on the diaphragmatic muscle.

Lung neoplasms

119 When suppressing an intractable cough in advanced lung cancer, and in the case of codeine, when seeking to give temporary relief from a persistent, non-productive cough in viral bronchitis.

120 Surgery is not effective because of the rapid dissemination of this tumour. However, systemic chemotherapy has improved the prognosis considerably.

121 Thoracotomy is indicated when
(a) there is no evidence of metastases;
(b) the growth does not involve the pleura, chest wall, trachea or other main structures;
(c) respiratory function is sufficient to tolerate lobectomy or pneumonectomy;
(d) the patient is otherwise fit for anaesthesia.

Pulmonary sarcoidosis

122 Usually for 1–2 years. Premature cessation of
     therapy leads to relapse.

Respiratory physiotherapy

123 Postural drainage, percussion and vibration. The
     yield of sputum may be increased by prior
     bronchodilator inhalation.

Alveolitis

124 With steroids. Prednisolone 20 mg/day is a
     reasonable starting dose but a higher dose will
     be required if the patient is very ill. Progress
     may be monitored using clinical and radio-
     logical features and serial measurements of
     transfer factor (Tl_{co}).

125 The response to steroids is unpredictable and
     spontaneous remissions also make it difficult to
     assess response. Approximately 50% of patients
     will appear to respond and in these cortico-
     steroids may need to be continued for several
     years until death, or less commonly a complete
     remission, occurs.

Bronchoscopy

126 Bronchoscopy provides a means for removal of
     a foreign body and for aspirating plugs of
     mucus that may be obstructing the larger
     airways.

Pneumothorax

127 Forty-eight hours after air has stopped bubbling
     out of the tube and chest X-rays show full
     expansion of the lung the chest drain is clamped.
     If the lung is still fully expanded 24 hours
     later the drain can be removed.

Hiatus hernia

128   Severe oesophagitis or an oesophageal stricture.

Peptic ulceration

129   Give up smoking, avoid alcohol, avoid aspirin and eat frequent small meals. Take steps to avoid stressful situations.

130   When taken at least ½ hour before food, the compound forms a tenacious coating over an ulcerated surface without influencing gastric acidity.

131   Carbenoxolone is an extract of liquorice which increases the lifespan of the gastric mucosal cells and the protective effect of gastric mucus. It causes sodium retention and potassium wasting (an aldosterone-like effect).

132   It is very important not to overlook malignancy. Early malignant ulcers may give an initial impression of healing with this form of therapy.

133   Cimetidine occasionally causes diarrhoea and rashes. Confusion has also been reported but this is only likely in the presence of renal or hepatic failure.

134   The equivalent of neutralizing approximately 150 mmol of HCl 1 h and 3 h after meals and at bedtime. For a weak antacid like magnesium trisilicate this could mean 600 cc of antacid mixture per day, which is impracticable.

135   Iron, tetracyclines, chlorpromazine, and mexiletine.

136   Provided that bleeding appears to have stopped and there is no imminent prospect of surgery, a regular diet may be given. Food, particularly protein, acts as a buffer.

137   Calcium in milk stimulates gastrin production thus increasing the secretion of acid.

138   Warfarin, diazepam, phenytoin and aminophyl-
      line.

Gall bladder disease

139   Diarrhoea is the normal side effect of cheno-
      deoxycholic acid and usually limits the dose
      that can be given.

140   Ampicillin, cephalosporins, cephamycins and
      metronidazole attain therapeutic levels in bile.
      Erythromycin does also, but is not effective
      against the usual Gram-negative pathogens
      found in acute cholecystitis.

Portal hypertension

141   The maximum rate at which ascitic fluid can be
      reabsorbed is 700-900 ml/24 h. If negative fluid
      balance exceeds this, then the lost fluid is com-
      ing from other compartments. If there is deple-
      tion of the circulating volume then renal
      perfusion will fall and renal failure (hepatorénal
      failure) may ensue.

142   Removal of ascites and reduction of intra-
      abdominal pressure may allow rapid transuda-
      tion into the peritoneal cavity with a fall in
      circulating volume. Removal of ascites may de-
      plete sodium as well as water, and ensuing
      hypotension may cause renal failure or precipi-
      tate encephalopathy in chronic liver disease.

Oesophageal varices

143   This dose of vasopressin, which lowers portal
      venous pressure by reducing splanchnic arterial
      flow, is effective for up to 1 hour. Following
      vasopressin administration abdominal pain and
      evacuation of the bowels indicate that the pre-
      paration is active. Their absence suggests inert
      hormone. Coronary vasoconstriction also
      occurs, making the drug hazardous in patients
      with ischaemic heart disease.

144   The gastric balloon should be filled with 200–
      300 cc of air. The pressure in the oesophageal
      balloon should be in the range 20–30 mmHg,
      a little above expected portal vein pressure.

Malabsorption

145 Coeliac disease is a cause of malabsorption.
Folic acid and iron deficiency are common and
there may also be deficiency of vitamins A, D,
K and B_{12}. All of these vitamins, and iron,
should be given.

146 Tetracycline should be given for the first 10
days of every month indefinitely in a dose of
250 mg four times daily for an adult.

Drug absorption

147 The absorption of all of these drugs is reduced
by the presence of food in the stomach.

Inflammatory bowel disorders

148 Sulphasalazine sometimes has a slight prophylactic effect in mild to moderate Crohn's
disease.

149 In Crohn's disease azathioprine has a steroid-
sparing effect and also contributes to maintaining a remission. By contrast, azathioprine
is little used in ulcerative colitis since surgery is
more readily resorted to when corticosteroids
fail to control the disease.

150 Prednisolone retention enemas (20 mg prednisolone in 100 cc) or hydrocortisone foam
(10% strength) are both effective. Oral prednisolone is needed if topical steroids fail.

151 In type I hypersensitivity reactions to foodstuffs
sodium cromoglycate can prevent symptoms.

Diarrhoea

152 Loperamide. It is usually given in 2 mg doses up
to a total of 16 mg/day.

Constipation

153 Fibre-containing preparations are classified as
bulk-forming agents and include miller's bran,

ispaghula husk and methylcellulose.

154 Phenolphthalein is colourless in acid urine but turns red if the urine is made alkaline.

155 In the treatment of hepatic encephalopathy.

156 Straining at stool should be prevented following myocardial infarction, subarachnoid haemorrhage, neurosurgery and when haemorrhoids or varicose veins are present.

Abdominal sepsis

157 Gentamicin 80 mg 8-hourly for 24 h plus metronidazole 500 mg 8-hourly for 24 h. An alternative is cefoxitin 1 g 8-hourly for 24 h. The first dose should be given at the time of operation.

Liver and Pancreatic Disorders

Hepatic encephalopathy

158 Thiazide and loop diuretics (frusemide, bumetanide), corticosteroids and carbenoxolone, all tend to cause potassium depletion.

159 No antiemetic is without risk but antihistamines are less risky than metoclopramide, and metoclopramide is less risky than prochlorperazine or other phenothiazines.

160 Most of the drug is excreted by the kidneys, with less than 40% being metabolized by a normal liver. In liver failure a smaller percentage will be metabolized by the liver but the half-life will not be very much prolonged.

161 In the initial stage of treatment the diet should contain no protein. Subsequently 20–40 g of protein can be introduced and more may be tolerated thereafter.

162 Branched-chain amino acids are important precursors in the production of neurotransmitters in the brain, but their blood level is typically reduced in most acute or chronic liver disease.

Administration in hepatic encephalopathy is on the grounds that correction of reduced levels of neurotransmitters may improve the encephalopathy.

163 In the treatment of hepatic encephalopathy lactulose lowers faecal pH. A fall in blood ammonia levels accompanies this. The mechanism of this effect is debated.

Viral hepatitis

164 None of these measures have been found to significantly benefit patients with acute hepatitis A, which is the cause of this boy's illness. It is reasonable for patients to avoid foods which worsen their nausea or anorexia, but fat restriction is not indicated. Vitamins are only necessary in malnourished cases. Rest is necessary only to the extent that the patient desires. Steroids are not of value in acute viral hepatitis.

165 Patients and staff involved with hemodialysis, liver disease, haemophilia and oncology. Dentists should also be vaccinated.

The vaccine has been prepared predominantly with serum from homosexuals who are the main sufferers from the acquired immunodeficiency syndrome (AIDS). Theoretically there is a possibility of the vaccine being contaminated with the transmissible agent causing AIDS.

Chronic active HBsAg negative hepatitis

166 In chronic active HBsAg negative hepatitis steroids will prolong life without preventing the ultimate development of cirrhosis. (Prednisolone rather than prednisone should be used).

167 Allopurinol. A quarter to a third of the usual dose of azathioprine is indicated if allopurinol cannot be stopped.

Cholestasis

168 Digoxin is bound by cholestyramine with a consequent reduction in absorption. The same

is true of paracetamol. The action of warfarin tends to be potentiated due to malabsorption of vitamin K which is fat-soluble.

Drugs and liver disease

169 In chronic hepatitis the oral contraceptive should not be used but in acute viral hepatitis it is not contraindicated. In women who have developed pregnancy cholestasis the oral contraceptive can be expected to cause cholestasis.

170 Streptomycin, ethambutol and cycloserine are not usually hepatotoxic.

171 Corticosteroid-induced fluid retention is more common in liver disease, as is the fluid retention and gastrointestinal bleeding due to NSAIDs.

Wilson's disease

172 Life-long.

Pancreatic disease

173 Aprotinin is a polypeptide which inhibits trypsin and also, to a lesser extent, fibrinolysis. After a loading dose of 500,000 units by slow IV injection, 200,000 units are given every 4 hours.

174 Pancreatin is inactivated by gastric acidity. Simultaneous administration of cimetidine will reduce gastric acid production.

Renal Disorders

Glomerulonephritis

175 Infertility, more commonly in males, and an increased incidence of bladder carcinoma.

176 Minimal change disease is virtually always sensitive to steroids while approximately half of all cases of membranous glomerulonephritis

will respond. Other forms such as focal sclerosing, mesangio-capillary and IgA nephropathy are not usually sensitive to steroids.

177 Plasmapheresis has been found useful in some cases of the following: SLE, rapidly progressive glomerulonephritis, haemolytic–uraemic syndrome, myasthenia gravis. Sporadic success in over a hundred other conditions has been reported. In Waldenstrom's macroglobulinaemia and multiple myeloma it is an effective treatment for hyperviscosity.

178 In the presence of clinical disease (proteinuria, nephrotic syndrome) membranous changes on renal biopsy are an indication for prednisone (in a high dose initially then tapering to a low maintenance dose). In the presence of mesangial proliferation, azathioprine may be added to steroids and must be added if proliferation is diffuse and renal function deteriorating. In rapidly progressive glomerulonephritis, steroids and cyclophosphamide are indicated possibly with methylprednisolone pulse therapy and plasma exchange.

Nephrotic syndrome

179 Anticoagulation or fibrinolytic therapy. Recovery of renal function may be good if the area of venous infarction is limited.

180 Albumin infusions.

Renal tubular acidosis

181 The correct dose is that which brings blood pH and serum potassium levels back to normal.

182 Indomethacin reduces glomerular filtration rate.

Urinary tract infection

183 Erythromycin reaches good levels in the prostate. Nearly all other antibiotics do not.
    Measures to prevent recurrent cystitis include bladder emptying within 15 minutes of intercourse, avoidance of spermicidal creams

that may cause urethral irritation, nightly
cleansing of the perineum and introitus with a
bactericidal solution and single-dose antibiotic therapy at night.

Renal stones

184   The diuretic hydrochlorothiazide. The usual
dose is 50 mg daily orally.

185   Yes, and so are gooseberries, raspberries, plums
and rhubarb.

186   Pyridoxine, in a dose of 800 mg daily.

Renal artery stenosis

187   Percutaneous renal angioplasty. In this technique a catheter with a specially designed low-
volume, high-pressure inflatable balloon at the
tip is passed into the stenosed renal artery
under fluoroscopic control. Balloon inflation
dilates the stenotic segment.

Renal failure

188   One gram of sodium chloride contains 17 millimoles of sodium; 1 gram of sodium bicarbonate
contains 12 millimoles of sodium.

189   Administration of phosphate binders reduces
phosphate absorption and with full doses it is
possible to bring phosphate levels back to normal. Aluminium hydroxide is the most commonly used compound; calcium carbonate is
another. Unfortunately many preparations are
unpalatable and lack of compliance is common.
A typical adult daily requirement would be
3–6 grams in divided doses.

190   None. Chloramphenicol is metabolized normally in all degrees of renal failure.

191   In uraemia, hepatic acetylation is impaired.

192   Tetracyclines, with the exception of doxycy-
cline, cause a deterioration in renal function in

the presence of renal failure. Nalidixic acid excretion into the urine is delayed in renal failure and it may fail to reach therapeutic concentrations. Nitrofurantoin accumulates when glomerular filtration rate is less than 20 ml/min, with an increased incidence of side effects, particularly peripheral neuropathy.

193 In uraemia, metoclopramide has a prolonged half-life, due to an enterohepatic circulation, and there is an appreciable incidence of extra-pyramidal side effects such as facial dyskinesia. Other phenothiazines should also be used with caution.

194 The only resort is to measure drug levels in the plasma, and adjust doses to keep the drug level in the therapeutic range. The therapeutic range for digoxin usually lies between 0.8 and 2 μg/l. Gentamicin peak levels should not exceed 10 mg/l and trough levels should not be greater than 2 mg/l.

195 A large fluid intake can prevent the formation of mixed renal stones in patients susceptible to stone formation and will slowly dissolve cystine stones. In cystitis, dilution of the bacterial pop-ulation with a large urine flow can be sufficient to flush out the infection. Antibiotics will also be diluted, however.

196 Alkalinization of the urine, often with 100 millimoles of sodium bicarbonate daily (100 millimoles = 8 grams) in conjunction with a high fluid intake will dissolve both uric acid and cystine stones.
   Alkalinization of the urine, usually with potassium citrate, is also traditional treatment (although dangerous in the presence of renal failure) for the relief of dysuria due to infection.

197 Foods containing above-average amounts of potassium include dates, raisins, apricots, carrots, chips, bananas, and orange juice.

198 Desferrioxamine. This chelating agent is better known for its capacity to bind iron in iron poisoning and states of iron overload, e.g. chronic haemolytic anaemias such as thalas-saemia major.

Haemodialysis

199 One tablet of ferrous gluconate daily and 1 mg of folic acid daily is usually adequate.

200 Regional heparinization, which means that the heparinization is confined to the dialyser. Blood returning from the dialyser to the patient is treated with protamine sulphate to reverse the heparin effect.

Peritoneal dialysis

201 The young, the elderly and diabetics.

Renal transplantation

202 Prednisone is reduced to 20 mg daily during the first few months and if graft function remains stable may be subsequently reduced further, preferably to an alternate-day regimen. Azathioprine should be given at 2–3 mg/kg/day or as much as the blood count will tolerate if graft function is critical.

203 Tremor, gingival hypertrophy and hirsutism can occur with long term cyclosporin A therapy.

204 The goal of this form of aspirin therapy should be to poison the platelets without blocking the synthesis of prostacyclin. Experimental evidence to date suggests that only a very low dose is needed, e.g. 50 mg every 48 h.

Endocrine Disorders

Pituitary disorders

205 Patients with prolactin-secreting microadenomas without evidence of suprasellar extension should be treated with bromocriptine. Those with large tumours should have surgery or radiotherapy followed by bromocriptine.

206 ACTH deficiency requires replacement doses of hydrocortisone or synthetic glucocorticoids. Mineralocorticoid supplements are not neces-

sary. TSH deficiency necessitates treatment with L-thyroxine. Growth hormone supplements are only required in GH-deficient children whose epiphyses are not fused. In males, androgen deficiency should be treated by depot injections of testosterone esters. Females with oestrogen deficiency may be treated with a cyclical oestrogen – progestogen combination.

207 Yttrium-90 implantation in the pituitary may be effective where the disease originates from the pituitary. Otherwise bilateral adrenalectomy following preparation of the patient for surgery is necessary.

Hyperthyroidism

208 Agranulocytosis occurs in about 1 case in 1000. It may lead to fatal infection. Presenting features include sore throat, furunculosis or fever, and patients should be warned to stop the antithyroid drugs and to report for a white cell count should these symptoms develop. Fortunately this agranulocytosis is usually reversible, but patients who develop it should avoid all further use of antithyroid drugs.

209 Propranolol is useful for achieving rapid control of thyrotoxic symptoms while waiting for antithyroid drugs or radioiodine to take effect. It is also useful in preparing patients for thyroid surgery. It is not advisable to use propranolol for long-term control of hyperthyroidism as it seldom controls symptoms fully and it has a low remission rate.

210 Iodide, usually given in the form of a supersaturated solution of potassium iodide, should be reserved for the treatment of thyroid storm or for preparing the thyroid gland for surgery. The dose used is one or two drops tid. Larger doses may produce toxic effects such as skin rash, enlargement of salivary glands and gynaecomastia.

211 Weight gain and slowing of pulse rate are useful signs of response. The serum T_4 should be checked at least once a month and it is a reasonably good guide to adequacy of therapy. The thyroid gland may shrink if the underlying disease remits. Increase in the size of the gland

may occur due to worsening of hyperthyroidism (low TSH) or drug-induced hypothyroidism (high TSH).

212 Hyperthyroidism due to toxic adenomas does not usually remit spontaneously and radio-iodine or surgery is usually needed.

213 Large doses of carbimazole (60–120 mg/day) or propylthiouracil (600–1200 mg/day) should be given orally or via nasogastric tube to inhibit hormone synthesis. An iodide preparation should be given in order to inhibit hormone release – e.g. supersaturated potassium iodide 5–10 drops 8-hourly orally. Propranolol 1.5 mg IV or 40–80 mg orally given every 6 h will block the peripheral effects of hyperthyroidism. Finally dexamethasone 2 mg 6-hourly should be given to inhibit tissue production of T_3 from T_4 and to treat any relative adrenal insufficiency which may accompany severe thyrotoxicosis.

214 Tarsorrhaphy should be considered when prop-tosis is so severe that the eye is exposed during sleep. High-dose corticosteroids may be of benefit in some cases but an effect is unlikely if there is no evidence of improvement after 1 month of therapy. Orbital decompression is indicated when corneal ulceration or loss of visual acuity occur.

215 The patient should be made euthyroid before surgery. This usually requires a 1–2-month course of antithyroid drugs. 1–2 weeks of iodide therapy before surgery reduces the vascularity of the thyroid gland and increases its firmness. Preparation using propranolol alone is risky as this drug has a short-lived effect and omission of one or more doses may be followed by a thyroid storm or severe exacerbation of hyperthyroidism.

216 It is difficult to predict the dose of ^{131}I required in each individual case. Usually 3–4 mCi are used initially in Graves' disease. If the con-dition is not controlled after about 4 months a repeat dose may be given. There is a steadily rising incidence of hypothyroidism each year after its use and thus patients require follow-up for life. ^{131}I takes 2–3 months to produce a therapeutic effect and thus antithyroid drugs

or propanolol should not be prematurely discontinued while awaiting this effect.

217 Antithyroid drugs cross the placenta and carry a risk of inducing goitre or cretinism in the fetus. Thus the smallest dose which produces a near-normal metabolic state in the mother should be used. The aim should be to maintain the maternal serum T_4 just above the upper limit of normal. The best laboratory tests are either free serum T_4 or free thyroxine index because of the increased thyroid hormone binding capacity of the maternal serum.

Hypothyroidism

218 Precipitation of angina or arrhythmias is a potentially serious complication of treatment and in such patients gradual replacement of thyroid hormone should commence with a dose of 25–50 μg of L-thyroxine per day. The dose may be increased by 25–50 μg at intervals of about 2 weeks until the full replacement dose is reached.

219 Hypoventilation and CO_2 retention may require assisted ventilation. Hypotension should be treated with isotonic fluids. Hypothermia should be treated by exposure to room temperature. IV dextrose may be required for hypoglycaemia. CNS depressants should be avoided and infection should be treated.

Thyroid nodules

220 Opinions vary on this question. Some authorities advise radionuclide scan initially in order to distinguish hot from cold nodules. Cold nodules are then further evaluated by ultrasound scanning in order to distinguish solid from cystic lesions. Solid cold nodules are then excised whereas fine-needle aspiration is carried out on cystic lesions and these are only excised if cytology shows malignant change. Other clinicians advise excision biopsy of all cold nodules as there is a small risk that fine-needle aspiration cytology may miss malignant change.

Addison's disease

221   One litre of normal saline with 5% dextrose should be given IV over 1 h. Several litres of saline may be required in the first 24 h in order to control sodium deficiency. Hydrocortisone 100 mg 6-hourly IV should be given for 24–48 h, after which it may be given orally and gradually reduced to the maintenance dose of 20–30 mg/day. Maintenance therapy should include 0.05 mg fludrocortisone daily for its mineralocorticoid effect.

Corticosteroids

222   For major surgery 100 mg hydrocortisone should be given IM with premedication, to be followed by 100 mg 6-hourly for 3 days or until the patient is eating. Thereafter the dose may be tapered to the standard maintenance dose over a few days. Patients with acute medical illness should take approximately twice their normal daily steroid dose during the acute period and then taper rapidly to their usual daily dosage.

223   H_2 blockers should not be prescribed routinely for patients on steroids alone but are often given to those taking other ulcerogenic medications such as aspirin in addition to steroids. If a 'steroid ulcer' develops in a patient on steroids and it is necessary to continue the steroids, ulcer therapy should be given. However, development of complications such as bleeding or perforation makes discontinuation of steroid therapy strongly advisable.

Conn's syndrome

224   A potassium-sparing diuretic is indicated. Although spironolactone is an aldosterone antagonist, side effects with spironolactone are not uncommon. Of the two alternatives, amiloride and triamterene, amiloride does not require hepatic activation and is the drug of choice.

Phaeochromocytoma

225 Twenty-four hour urine total metanephrines is
the test least likely to give a false-positive result
due to dietary or medicinal contamination.
   Thiazides, propranolol, clonidine, hydralazine and phentolamine and phenoxybenzamine
can be given without risk of diagnostic error.

226 Careful cardiovascular monitoring, including
continuous intra-arterial blood pressure monitoring, is necessary.
   IV alpha and beta blockers are used to
control blood pressure and arrhythmias. The
short-acting vasodilator sodium nitroprusside
may also be useful in this situation. Careful
attention to volume replacement is essential
since patients with a phaeochromocytoma
typically have a reduced circulating volume
and are vulnerable to postoperative hypotension.

Hypogonadism

227 IM administration of a long-acting ester of
testosterone such as testosterone oenanthate
250 mg every 2–4 weeks is the treatment of
choice. The dose interval should be adjusted
so that androgen withdrawal symptoms are
prevented between injections. An occasional
side effect is polycythaemia and it is therefore
important to measure the haematocrit every
3–4 months.

Amenorrhoea

228 Clomiphene is effective in producing ovulation
in cases of polycystic ovary disease and also in
cases with amenorrhoea following the use of
oral contraceptives, in psychogenic
amenorrhoea and amenorrhoea persisting after
weight regain. Although successful in inducing
ovulation, it is less often followed by pregnancy. Side effects include ovarian cyst formation, hot flushes and blurring of vision. It is
contraindicated in women with a history of
liver disease.

Hirsutism

229   Dysfunctional hirsutism occurs in cases lacking
a clearly demonstrable organic or biochemical
lesion. These may respond well to the anti-
androgen cyproterone acetate. This drug must
be avoided in pregnancy as it may interfere
with sexual differentiation of the male fetus.

Metabolic Disorders

Diabetes mellitus

230   The American Diabetes Association diet aims
to reduce fat content to 25–35% of total
calories and to provide 40–55% of calories
as carbohydrate and 12–24% as protein.
Rapidly absorbed sugars should be avoided
and carbohydrates provided instead in the
form of leguminous foods, rice or pasta.
Excessive restriction of calories should not
be used in managing insulin-dependent or
pregnant diabetics.

231   No. The majority of diabetics are poorly informed about their disease. Doctors caring
for diabetics must inform themselves about
methods and resources for education of their
patients. A team approach to this problem is
probably best and it should involve cooper-
ation between the doctor, the nurse and the
dietician.

232   Optimal diabetic control is obtained by giving
insulin twice daily. Generally two-thirds of the
total daily dose should be given before break-
fast and the remaining third before the evening
meal. Each of the injections should consist of
approximately two-thirds intermediate-acting
and one-third short-acting (neutral, soluble)
insulin. A total dose of approximately 30 units
of insulin per day is a reasonable starting dose
for a non-obese adult. Further adjustments
should be based on the blood glucose profile
and clinical improvement.

233   More severe reactions may be treated by giving
1 mg of glucagon IM or SC by relatives or IV
if medical personnel are available to administer

it. This should be followed by oral glucose or a meal following recovery of consciousness. If glucagon is not available, or if the patient fails to respond to it within 10–15 min, 20–40 ml of 20–50% dextrose may be given IV. This has the advantage of causing phlebitis in some cases but should not be withheld when the situation is serious.

234 The patient is kept fasting and the usual morning insulin dose is omitted on the day of operation. Blood glucose may be controlled by a glucose/insulin IV infusion during surgery and the postoperative period. The usual doses are 0.5–2 units of soluble insulin plus 5–10 grams of glucose (as 5% dextrose) per hour. Blood glucose should be estimated immediately before surgery and thereafter 4-hourly with appropriate adjustments in insulin dose until the patient can resume eating normally and take his usual insulin regime.

235 The commonest cause of immunologically mediated insulin resistance is the development of high levels of anti-insulin IgG antibody in patients on insulin therapy. Treatment with high doses of steroids (prednisolone 60 mg/day) may successfully reduce insulin requirements.

236 Those with liver disease or renal impairment, and alcoholics, are particularly prone to develop hypoglycaemia. Chlorpropamide should not be used in the elderly because of its long half-life. It is also contraindicated in cases where a full-blown episode of ketoacidosis has occurred in the past.

237 Probably via a number of mechanisms including a degree of intestinal malabsorption, reduction in glucose production by the liver, and by increasing peripheral uptake of glucose by making more receptors available for insulin.

238 The average fluid deficit in adults with diabetic ketoacidosis is 3–5 litres. One litre of normal saline should be run in over the first ½ hour. A further 1–2 litres should be given during the next 2–3 hours and the remainder of the deficit plus the continuing losses should be replaced during the remainder of the first 24 hours. Half-strength saline should be used if hyperna-

traemia is present, and when the blood glucose
falls to about 12 mmol/l, 5% dextrose in water
should be used.

239   Serum potassium should be estimated 2-hourly
during initial therapy. If it is ⩾6.5 mmol/l no
potassium should be given ·with the first litre
of IV fluid. Thereafter 20–40 mmol of potassium per litre of fluid is usually required to
maintain normokalaemia.

240   When the patient's general condition has improved and blood pH has returned to normal
and the blood glucose has fallen to about
12 mmol/l it is reasonable to give insulin via
the SC route on a 4-hourly basis. Even though
the blood glucose level may have fallen to
normal, the insulin infusion should be continued as long as acidosis or ketosis are present.

241   If the patient is hypotensive or if the plasma
sodium is under 150 mmol/l normal saline may
be used. Otherwise half normal may be used.
Large volumes of fluid are usually required
(1–2 litres in the first hour). Therapy should be
monitored with a CVP line.

242   Treatment should include discontinuation of
biguanide therapy. Large volumes of isotonic
bicarbonate should be given IV so as to raise
the blood pH above 7. Haemodialysis or peritoneal dialysis may be required in order to
eliminate excessive amounts of sodium.

243   (a) Reduction of oedema by destroying leak-
ing blood vessels.
(b) Prevention and elimination of new vessel
formation by destroying areas of abnormal
avascular retina.
(c) Destruction of abnormal blood vessels lo-
cated in the pre-retinal area.

244   A fasting blood glucose of 5 mmol/l and a
postprandial level of 6.5 mmol/l, while avoiding
hypoglycaemia, should be the objective of good
control. This degree of control certainly carries
a risk of maternal hypoglycaemia but fortunately the fetus seems to tolerate this well.

245   Biguanides are more liable to cause lactic
acidosis in the presence of renal impairment.

Chlorpropamide is largely excreted by the kidney and is more likely to produce hypoglycaemia in patients with renal failure.

Hyperlipidaemia

246   Cholestyramine interferes with absorption of digoxin and warfarin, thiazides and thyroxine, all of which should be given either 1 hour before or 4 hours after administration of cholestyramine. Absorption of fat-soluble vitamins is also impaired and vitamin supplements are indicated in patients on cholestyramine. They are best given at night.

Inborn errors of metabolism

247   Barbiturates, sulphonamides, oral contraceptives and sulphonylureas. Dieting to lose weight may also precipitate an acute attack.

248   Vomiting may be controlled with chlorpromazine or metoclopramide. Aspirin, paracetamol, dihydrocodeine, pethidine and morphine may be used for pain relief. Diazepam and sodium valproate can be safely used to treat convulsions. Propranolol may be used to treat hypertension or tachycardia. Penicillin and tetracycline are safe antibiotics and neostigmine may be used for constipation.

249   The clinical and biochemical picture is that of erythropoietic protoporphyria, an autosomal dominant disorder which can occur at any age. Most cases respond to β-carotene 120–180 mg daily. The resulting carotenaemia causes yellowing of the skin but this may be modified by adding canthaxanthin.

250   There appear to be two variants of homocystinuria. One variety responds well to pyridoxine 600 mg daily. The other type requires a low-methionine diet with cystine, vitamin and mineral supplements.

Disorders of Mineral and Bone Metabolism

Hypocalcaemia

251 Serum calcium levels should be checked
regularly in order to avoid the development
of hypercalcaemia. If the active vitamin D preparations such as 1α-hydroxycholecalciferol are
used, dosage should be increased very slowly.
These agents do have the advantages of faster
onset of action and shorter half-life activity.
Toxicity is more rapidly reversible should it
occur.

252 Alkalosis may be due to persistent vomiting, in
which case IV normal saline is an effective
treatment. If alkalosis is secondary to administration of alkalis, these should be stopped and
in addition oral ammonium chloride may be
needed. Alkalosis secondary to hysterical
hyperventilation can be effectively controlled
by getting the patients to rebreathe their own
expired air from a bag.

Hypercalcaemia

253 Tumour irradiation or chemotherapy may be
effective in controlling hypercalcaemia due to
ectopic ACTH production. When hypercalcaemia is due to bone secondaries or multiple myeloma, prednisolone in doses of up to
30 mg/day may be valuable. In some cases
NSAIDs are effective.

254 Steroids, calcitonin, mithramycin and phosphate supplementation may be useful, but
their use must be guided by clinical circumstances.

255 Oral cellulose phosphate reduces calcium
absorption. Unfortunately the absorption of
oxalates tends to increase.

Disorders of phosphate and magnesium metabolism

256 Magnesium sulphate should be given in the
form of a 10% solution, 1–2 g over 10–15 min.

This should be followed by IM injections of 1 g
6-hourly until clinical recovery occurs and
normal serum levels are restored.

257 Mild cases may be treated by oral administration of a phosphate salt. More severe hypophosphataemia may require parenteral therapy.
Note that calcium and phosphorus solutions
should not be combined in the same infusion.

Metabolic bone disease

258 Calcium supplements (1–2 g/day) and up to
50,000 IU of vitamin D daily may be necessary
to produce bone healing. Treatment should be
monitored by checking serum calcium and
alkaline phosphatase levels regularly.

259 Diphosphonates may relieve bone pain in
Paget's disease and they have the great advantage of oral administration. Disodium etidro-
nate (EHDP) does not appear to heal osteolytic
lesions in every case and may occasionally cause
osteomalacia. Dichloromethylene diphosphon-
ate (Cl_2MDP) appears less likely to cause this
side effect.

260 Steroid-induced osteopenia appears to be due
to a combination of osteoporosis due to direct
inhibition of the formation of bone, and
osteitis resulting from hyperparathyroidism
secondary to reduced calcium absorption.
Patients on steroids should be encouraged to
be as active as possible and the steroid dose
should be kept to the minimum possible.
Supplements of calcium and vitamin D may
help by suppressing secondary hyperparathyroidism.

261 Administration of oestrogens following the
menopause does reduce the development of
osteoporosis but this treatment carries a risk
of endometrial cancer and thrombosis. The
former problem may be prevented by using
an oestrogen combined with a progestogen
and administering the combination on a
cyclical basis. However because of the danger
some prefer to confine this form of prophylaxis to women who have an early menopause
(under 40).

Disorders of Water and Electrolyte Metabolism

Disorders of water metabolism

262 Restriction of fluid intake to less than 1 litre/24 hours is effective if it can be tolerated. Democycline 600 mg bd is an effective alternative.

263 Chlorpropamide, tolbutamide, vincristine, cyclophosphamide and morphine.

Disorders of sodium metabolism

264 One litre of 10% dextrose water followed by 1 litre of 5% dextrose water/0.45% saline, each litre having 20 mmol KCl added, and each litre to run over 12 hours. Considerably larger quantities will be required when abnormal losses occur.

265 Administration of fluids such as dextrose water, which contains no sodium, to patients who are both water- and sodium-depleted may precipitate severe hyponatraemia with confusion, weakness, vomiting and even seizures. Thus it is necessary to use sodium-containing fluids such as normal saline in most cases of volume depletion. However, administration of excessive salt should be avoided. This may be achieved by monitoring neck veins, lung bases, CVP and serum sodium.

266 Steroids, ACTH, NSAIDs, oral contraceptives, androgens and carbenoxolone.

Disorders of potassium metabolism

267 This is a less common toxic effect of diuretics. It is characterized by sodium depletion in association with persistent oedema. Clinical features include apathy, vomiting, hypotension and tachycardia. Biochemical features include elevated blood urea and hyponatraemia. Treatment includes sodium replacement, preferably orally, to avoid additional fluid administration. Occasionally administration of small amounts of IV hypertonic saline may be of benefit, e.g.

(200 ml of 5% saline given slowly).

268   In situations where serum K^+ is less than 2 mmol/l or when ECG abnormalities or paralysis are present the maximum rate of potassium administration should not exceed 40 mmol/h and its concentration should not exceed 60 mmol/l. Administration of potassium at this rate is dangerous and the ECG should be monitored and the serum K^+ checked hourly.

269   A dose of 5–10 ml of 10% calcium gluconate should be given IV over about 2 min. This protects the heart from the toxic effects of hyperkalaemia, but its effect is short-lived. A dose of 44 mmol of $NaHCO_3$ may also be given IV over 5 min; this causes K^+ to move into cells. A dextrose insulin infusion should also be given as it has a similar effect. The above measures will improve the acute situation but in addition a cation exchange resin should be used to rid the body of excessive potassium. Haemodialysis is effective if the above measures fail.

270   Renal impairment. Concomitant administration of captopril also increases the risk of hyperkalaemia and is therefore contraindicated when potassium-sparing diuretics are used.

Acid–base disturbances

271   The reversal of mild metabolic acidosis by a normal saline solution is due to the ability of the kidney to reclaim more bicarbonate ions from the ultrafiltrate in the proximal tubule with the extra sodium available, while excreting more hydrogen ions in the distal tubule by virtue of the increased sodium–hydrogen ion exchange.

272   This biochemical picture suggests severe metabolic alkalosis due to prolonged vomiting and chloride replacement is indicated. If renal function is normal an infusion of isotonic saline will tend to reverse the alkalosis, but in view of its severity and the possibility of tetany occurring, an ammonium chloride/sodium chloride solution with potassium supplements is indicated.

273   By administration of chloride, either as the potassium or ammonium salt, depending on serum potassium levels. If potassium is given, care should be taken to ensure that potassium chloride, and not potassium bicarbonate, is what the patient actually receives.

Haematological Disorders

Aplastic anaemia

274   Idiosyncratic aplastic anaemia which is not dose-related and which is usually fatal. The incidence of this complication is about 1 : 25,000. It may occur many months after completion of the course of chloramphenicol. Because of this problem the use of chloramphenicol should be restricted to life-threatening disorders where it is the drug of choice, namely typhoid fever and *Haemophilus influenzae* meningitis.

275   Antineoplastic agents such as busulphan, methotrexate or daunorubicin, ionizing radiation and certain chemical and industrial agents such as benzene, trinitrotoluene, gamma-benzene hexachloride and organic arsenic compounds.

276   Soft toothbrushes should be used with care. A stool softener is indicated. Shaving should be with an electric razor. Salicylates and IM injections should be avoided because of the risk of haemorrhage. Skin should be kept scrupulously clean with antiseptic soap and carefully cleansed with iodine when venepuncture is required.

277   Bone marrow transplantation from a histocompatible donor (usually a sibling). Results are better in younger patients (i.e. under 30 years).

Iron deficiency anaemia

278   Nausea, diarrhoea, black stools. Antacids reduce nausea but also inhibit iron absorption. Despite the colour of the stools the guaiac test for occult blood is not affected, although the ortho-

toluidine test may give false-positive results.

279 IM iron dextran is a very painful injection and
may produce local staining of the tissues, fever,
headache, arthralgia, urticaria, nausea, vomiting
and rarely severe anaphylaxis. IV iron dextran
has the advantage of being painless and of
allowing replacement of the entire iron deficit,
but fatal anaphylaxis may occur within minutes
of commencing the infusion.

280 Patients with thalassaemia have a microcytic
anaemia but are commonly overloaded with
iron. Iron administration will only aggravate
this. Folic acid administration can precipitate
neurological damage in a patient with vitamin
B_{12} deficiency which has not been corrected.

Megaloblastic anaemia

281 Those with sickle-cell anaemia, myelofibrosis,
malabsorption or continuing dietary in-
adequacy.

282 Both hydroxocobalamin and cyanocobalamin
have B_{12} activity but hydroxocobalamin has
a longer half-life due to greater protein-binding.
It is therefore preferable for maintenance
therapy since an injection is required only every
2 or 3 months.
   Hypokalaemia may occur due to potassium
uptake into the red cell mass which rapidly
increases when B_{12} therapy is initiated in
pernicious anaemia.

283 The bone marrow may revert from a megaloblastic to a normoblastic morphology in as
little as 2 days. Reticulocytosis begins within
2–3 days and peaks about the sixth day. Serum
bilirubin and LDH levels fall quickly, and the
patient begins to feel better by about the third
day. The red cell count is usually back to
normal 1–2 months after starting therapy.

Thrombocytopenia

284 Four days is the average half-life. The aim of
platelet transfusion is to stop bleeding and
raise the platelet count by at least 50,000/mm^3.

Usually a transfusion of about 8 units of stored platelets or 4 units of fresh platelets will achieve this.

285 Life-threatening haemorrhage at initial presentation, failure to respond to high-dose steroid therapy, or recurrence after withdrawal of steroids; 80% of cases of ITP will recover with splenectomy. The 20% who do not, may benefit from further steroid treatment or immunosuppression with azathioprine or vincristine.

286 Quinine and quinidine are the best-documented ones and act by producing antiplatelet antibodies. Heparin, gold, phenlybutazone, oxyphenbutazone, indomethacin, co-trimoxazole and diuretics may also cause thrombocytopenia. Recovery usually follows withdrawal of the offending drug but platelet transfusions may be required for haemorrhage or severe thrombocytopenia. Steroids may help those cases with drug-induced antiplatelet antibodies.

287 TTP carries a very high mortality and heparin, steroids and splenectomy have been tried without much success. Plasmapheresis, antiplatelet agents (aspirin, dipyridamole), and prostacyclin, however, appear to be of benefit.

Haemolysis

288 Splenectomy should be carried out on all children with spherocytosis even if anaemia is mild, because of the risk of complications such as cholelithiasis and aplastic crises. Splenectomized children should receive polyvalent pneumococcal vaccine, and some authorities recommend prophylactic penicillin for some years following splenectomy.

289 Ingestion of fava beans, viral hepatitis, diabetic ketoacidosis and acute febrile illness such as pneumonia.

290 Methlydopa causes haemolysis by an unknown mechanism. Antibiotics including cephalothin and penicillin may cause antibody-induced haemolysis, but the dose of penicillin required to do this is in excess of 20 megaunits/day

given IV. Quinidine and chlorpropamide may cause haemolysis via an immune complex mechanism. Hydralazine and procainamide may cause an SLE-like reaction.

291 The patient's autoantibodies usually react with donor red cells, thus making cross-matching very difficult. Minor blood group sensitivity may occur and iron overload will follow repeated transfusion. Thus transfusion should be withheld unless anaemia is very severe.

292 The underlying disorder should be treated where possible. Steroids are not helpful, which is in contrast to their effect in warm antibody autoimmune haemolytic anaemia. Some patients improve on low-dose chlorambucil but the main therapeutic approach is avoidance of cold exposure by change in lifestyle. Daily folate supplements are indicated.

293 Haemolytic crises may be treated by low molecular weight dextran infusions and if transfusion is required, washed red cells must be used as plasma infusion may exacerbate haemolysis. Androgen therapy may help reduce haemolysis and folate or iron supplements may be required if there is deficiency of these substances. Oral anticoagulants may be useful in reducing thrombotic problems but heparin may actually increase haemolysis and should not be used.

294 The transfusion must be stopped immediately; 25 g of mannitol should be given IV over 5 min. Urine output should be kept at a level of at least 100 cc/hour by giving IV fluids. If acute renal failure supervenes it must be treated in the usual manner by careful fluid and electrolyte balance. If further transfusion is required compatibility must be ensured by careful cross-matching.

295 By giving methylene blue 1 mg/kg IV if the patient is symptomatic; 100% oxygen should be given until the methaemoglobin has been reduced to haemoglobin.

Coagulation disorders

296   Parenteral vitamin K (10–20 mg) takes 6–12 hours to restore vitamin K-dependent factors to normal. However, vitamin K is not effective in the presence of severe liver cell disease and in this situation, or when bleeding is severe, a fresh-frozen plasma infusion is required to rapidly restore the deficient clotting factors to normal.

297   In life-threatening situations the aim is to raise the patient's factor VIII levels to 100% of normal initially. Half of the initial dose of factor VIII may then be given 8-hourly for 2 days and 12-hourly for about 4 days following onset of haemorrhage. The following formula may be used to calculate the amount of factor VIII required:
Units factor VIII needed = plasma volume × (target factor VIII level – initial factor VIII level).
Plasma volume = 41 ml/kg bodyweight approximately.

298   Aspirin impairs platelet aggregation due to inhibition of thromboxane production via its effect on the cyclo-oxygenase system in the platelet prostaglandin pathway. Thus it leads to increased bleeding time and may precipitate bleeding in any patient whose coagulation system is already impaired. Thus no aspirin-containing preparations should be given to patients with coagulation defects.

299   Aspirin-like drugs should be avoided. Bleeding usually responds to fresh-frozen plasma infusion but platelet transfusion may be required due to the functional platelet defect. Both bleeding time (for platelet function) and factor VIII activity should be monitored.

300   The main approach is to treat the underlying condition of sepsis, shock or malignancy. Fresh-frozen plasma or platelets may be needed, but heparin is certainly not standard therapy even though it may have helped occasionally in some patients.

Haemoglobinopathies

301 Folic acid supplements. Avoid flying in un-
pressurized aircraft as hypoxia may precipitate
a vaso-occlusive crisis. However, the level of
pressure in a commercial aircraft may also be
insufficient to prevent a crisis.

302 Infection must be vigorously sought by culture
of blood and other fluids, and if present
prompt treatment with appropriate antibiotics
is indicated. *Pneumococcus* and *Salmonella* are
common pathogens in sickle-cell disease. Analgesics are very necessary but narcotics should
be avoided as far as possible because of the
risks of addiction, and salicylates may be contraindicated because of accompanying G6PD
deficiency. Adequate hydration is one of the
most important measures and IV treatment is
usually needed. Acidosis should be corrected
and oxygen given. Severe cases may require
exchange transfusion. Daily haemoglobin levels
and reticulocyte counts are essential to identify
the development of an aplastic crisis.

303 By early institution of a vigorous iron chelation
programme with desferrioxamine.

304 Two to four grams over 12 hours. Urinary excretion of ferrioxamine, the chelate, is enhanced
by oral ascorbic acid.

Myeloproliferative disorders

305 Myelosuppressive therapy for PRV may be of
two forms. Firstly radioactive phosphorus 3–5
mCi may be given by a single IV injection. A
second injection may be required if an adequate
response has not been obtained in 2 months.
This treatment usually produces a long-lasting
remission. Alternatively oral busulphan given
on a daily basis is equally effective. There is a
small increase in the incidence of leukaemia
years after giving either of these forms of
therapy, but this is far less important than the
risk of thrombotic complications if the PRV is
not adequately controlled.

306 Myelosuppressive therapy with busulphan may
be useful when the peripheral white cell count

is high or when splenomegaly is progressive and the marrow is cellular. Splenectomy should be considered when there is significant haemolysis not responding to steroids or when there is progressive splenomegaly causing discomfort. However, before undertaking splenectomy it is necessary to ensure there is haematopoiesis outside the spleen, i.e. that the marrow is cellular.

Malignant Disease

Chemotherapeutic agents

307 Cyclophosphamide is inactive until metabolized in the liver to phosphoramide. However, a second metabolic product, acrolein, causes the haemorrhagic cystitis. The toxic effect of acrolein may be inhibited by simultaneous administration of 2-mercaptoethane sulphonic acid (mesna).

308 Bone marrow depression and neurotoxicity. Vincristine is mainly neurotoxic and this effect is manifested by loss of tendon reflexes and paraesthesiae of feet and hands with eventual sensory loss and paralysis. Severe neurological damage can usually be avoided by stopping or reducing the drug at the first sign of toxicity.

309 The main toxic effect of *cis*-platinum is on the renal tubule, and it is essential to give vigorous hydration before, during and after administration of the drug. Other toxic effects include marrow depression, ototoxicity and vomiting.

Radiotherapy

310 Palliative radiotherapy is useful in treating tumour-induced superior mediastinal syndrome, raised intracranial pressure or spinal cord compression. In addition palliative radiotherapy may relieve obstruction of the gastrointestinal or genitourinary tracts due to malignant disease. It is also effective in relieving bone pain due to metastases.

Leukaemia

311 By a course of cranial irradiation and intrathecal methotrexate.

312 A complete remission is obtained in about 80% of patients. Unfortunately the median duration of remission is only about 18 months.

313 Busulphan 4–6 mg daily orally. Therapy must be monitored by regular white cell and platelet counts and should be stopped when the white cell count falls to 20,000/mm^3 as continued treatment below this level may cause fatal marrow hypoplasia.

314 Chlorambucil given orally is effective in reducing the peripheral blood lymphocyte count towards normal and it also reduces splenomegaly and lymphadenopathy. Steroids in high dosage (60 mg/day of prednisolone) rapidly shrink lymph nodes but increase the risk of infection and are best reserved for cases with problems such as haemolysis, marrow failure or thrombocytopenia. Irradiation of enlarged lymph nodes or spleen will also relieve symptoms.

Hodgkin's disease

315 Patients with stage I, II and IIIA disease. However, even within these groups if there is a large volume of disease in the mediastinum, if more than two nodal sites above the diaphragm are involved, or if the histological picture is of a lymphocyte-depleted type, prognosis can be improved by giving a course of chemotherapy prior to radiotherapy.

316 Acute non-lymphocytic leukaemia may occur in up to 5% of Hodgkin's cases treated with chemotherapy who are followed up for periods of 5–10 years.

Gynaecological malignancy

317 Patients with choriocarcinoma may be divided into good-prognosis and poor-prognosis types. The former include those with metastases confined to lungs or pelvis and serum β-HCG levels

below 40,000 mIU/ml before therapy and who are commenced on therapy within 4 months of the start of the disease. These respond well to single-agent therapy with methotrexate or dactinomycin.

Patients with more advanced disease have a worse prognosis and should receive combination chemotherapy with regimes such as MAC (methotrexate, actinomycin, chlorambucil). Radiotherapy may be required for cerebral metastases.

318 Initially, as much malignant tissue as possible should be excised, and in general a bilateral salpingo-oophorectomy and total hysterectomy is carried out when there is extensive disease. Once spread outside the ovaries has occurred adjuvant chemotherapy is usually indicated. Combinations of drugs such as bleomycin, vinblastine and *cis*-platinum appear to be effective in prolonging survival, but are quite toxic.

Testicular tumours

319 Surgery and radiation are also employed in treating malignant teratoma of the testis, but chemotherapy is frequently required also.

Patients should be monitored by regular chest X-ray, CT scan or ultrasound of retroperitoneal lymph nodes and estimation of the specific tumour markers alpha-fetoprotein and human chorionic gonadotrophin.

Breast cancer

320 A 1-year course of the cyclical CMF regime (cyclophosphamide, methotrexate, fluorouracil) is used in premenopausal women with one to three positive lymph nodes. Premenopausal women with more lymph node involvement receive vincristine and prednisolone in addition to CMF. Patients with positive oestrogen and progesterone receptors receive tamoxifen, an anti-oestrogen preparation, instead of or in addition to the above regime.

Cancer of the prostate

321 Bilateral orchidectomy and diethylstilboestrol
in the absence of cardiovascular disease. If
hormonal therapy fails chemotherapy with
monthly cycles of 5-fluorouracil, doxorubicin
and mitomycin-C may be tried.

Multiple myeloma

322 Blood and platelet count, serum and urine
M-protein levels, serum calcium and creatinine
should be checked regularly. Melphalan treatment should be continued until M-protein levels
show no further decrease providing undue bone
marrow depression does not occur. Steroids are
continued until hypercalcaemia is controlled.

Bone marrow transplantation

323 The recipient is immunosuppressed with large
doses of cyclophosphamide and/or total body
irradiation. This destroys the recipient's bone
marrow. Then approximately ½ litre of marrow
is aspirated from the iliac crest of the donor
and infused IV into the recipient. It takes
about 3 weeks for the transplanted marrow
to develop in the recipient and during this
period intensive support is required.

324 Cyclosporin A. This is a toxic drug which can
cause neurotoxicity, nephrotoxicity and
hepatotoxicity. It can also cause hirsutism.
Absorption via the oral route is very variable
and thus serum levels must be checked twice
weekly by radioimmunoassay. Cyclosporin A
does not reduce the incidence of graft versus
host disease, but it reduces its severity.

Immunosuppression and infection

325 An aminoglycoside such as gentamicin plus a
semisynthetic anti-pseudomonas penicillin such
as ticarcillin or carbenicillin should be commenced IV. A cephalosporin such as cefazolin
may be substituted for the semisynthetic
penicillin in patients allergic to penicillin.

Malignant pleural effusion

326 Pleural effusions due to tumour invasion should
be treated by drainage followed by injection of
a sclerosant such as nitrogen mustard or bleomycin into the pleural cavity. Chylous effusions
due to lymphatic obstruction should be treated
by radiotherapy to the affected lymphatics.

Rheumatological Disorders

Septic arthritis

327 This picture suggests gonococcal arthritis,
which accounts for about one-third of all acute
bacterial arthritis. Penicillin is normally the
drug of choice, but as the patient is allergic to
penicillin, erythromycin is an effective alternative. Tetracycline may also be used.

328 This is the picture of acute infectious arthritis
due to staphylococcal infection. High-dose IV
antibiotics such as nafcillin, flucloxacillin or
clindamycin should be started immediately.
The joint should initially be immobilized in a
half cast and then mobilized as soon as the pain
has abated. Repeated arthrocentesis and
cultures are indicated to remove inflammatory
material and monitor progress. Antibiotics
should be continued for at least 3 weeks.

329 Aspirate the effusion. Patients with rheumatoid
arthritis, especially those whose immunity is
suppressed by steroids, are at increased risk of
acute bacterial arthritis. The aspirated synovial
fluid must be examined for organisms by Gram
stain and culture and the white cell count of
the fluid must be determined. If the fluid is
purulent, antibiotics must be started immediately and in high dosage. If no organism is
visible on Gram stain, a combination of nafcillin and gentamicin should be effective as the
likely pathogens are staphylococci or Gram-
negative bacilli.

Rheumatoid arthritis

330 Firstly, the patient must return immediately

should untoward symptoms develop. Full blood count and urinalysis must be done monthly. Gold injections must be discontinued immediately if rashes, thrombocytopenia, pancytopenia, proteinuria or the nephrotic syndrome develop.

331 Proteinuria due to penicillamine is usually benign. It is due to immune complex deposition in the kidney. It will usually disappear after about 14 months, even if treatment is continued. Renal function must be monitored regularly and 24 hour urine protein should be checked 3-monthly. However, if oedema develops, penicillamine must be stopped, as the hypovolaemia associated with the nephrotic syndrome may lead to a reduced glomerular filtration rate and uraemia.

332 Steroids do not appear to alter the course of rheumatoid arthritis and they do not improve the extra-articular features of the disease. Thus their effect is mainly symptomatic and because of their serious side effects they are better avoided altogether in rheumatoid arthritis.

333 Azathioprine must be avoided in pregnancy as it is teratogenic. Great caution is required in patients with renal or hepatic insufficiency. The major side effect of azathioprine is bone marrow depression, and therapy must be monitored by monthly blood counts. Allopurinol reduces the metabolism of azathioprine and the dose of azathioprine should be reduced by at least 70% in patients on allopurinol.

Osteoarthritis

334 Reassurance of the patient that the disease is generally non-progressive and non-deforming. Measures to reduce mechanical stress on joints, such as rest periods during work and weight reduction, are useful. Physical therapy with measures such as heat may relieve pain and stiffness.

335 The long-term durability of this procedure is still uncertain, although it appears very good up to 15 years. Complications include loosening of the components and infection of the interface

between the methyl methacrylate cement holding the polyethylene acetabular cup in place and the underlying pelvic bone.

Seronegative arthropathies

336   Regular exercise, especially swimming, should be encouraged once pain has been controlled. The patient should sleep on a firm mattress without a pillow in order to lessen the chances of spinal fusion occurring in a bent position. Deep breathing and back exercises are also important.

337   No. Approximately 10% of adult asthmatics have aspirin sensitivity. Ingestion of aspirin-containing substances produces severe asthma which may even be fatal in these individuals. Asthmatics with nasal polyps or sinusitis are especially likely to be aspirin-sensitive.

Connective tissue disorders

338   Antimalarial drug therapy in SLE is most useful in the skin lesions of discoid lupus, but photo-sensitivity, other rashes, athralgia and pleuritis may also respond.

339   When life-threatening complications occur in SLE very large IV doses of steroid may be life-saving. Usually, 500 mg methyl prednisolone is given IV over ½ hour every 12 hours for up to 5 days, followed by a gradually tapering dose of oral steroids.

340   Hydralazine and procainamide. Women, especially those who are HLA-DR 4 positive and slow acetylators, are prone to drug-induced SLE.

341   Decreased bowel motility may lead to bacterial overgrowth and malabsorption. Therapy with broad-spectrum antibiotics such as tetracycline frequently improves the malabsorption.

342   High-dose steroids e.g. prednisolone 60 mg daily. If response is slow, cytotoxic therapy with azathioprine or cyclophosphamide should

be added. If these fail, it may be necessary to resort to plasma exchange.

343 This clinical picture is very suggestive of poly-myalgia rheumatica with additional features of giant cell arteritis. He should immediately be commenced on 60 mg of prednisolone per day in order to prevent blindness. Bilateral temporal artery biopsy (2.5 cm on each side) should be done within a day or two of start-ing steroids. The dose of steroids may gradu-ally be tapered while monitoring the ESR. A maintenance dose may be required for years.

Gout and pseudogout

344 Allopurinol may precipitate an acute attack of gout during the initial months of therapy. Thus a prophylactic course of colchicine should be used for the first 3 months. Allo-purinol inhibits the enzyme mono-oxygenase, and this potentiates the effect of warfarin, cyclophosphamide, mercaptopurine and azathioprine, the dosages of which should therefore be reduced.

345 Stop the allopurinol as it is probably causing the rash and fever. Alternative but less effec-tive drugs are probenecid and sulphinpyrazone, which are uricosuric preparations. They should not be used in patients with urolithiasis.

346 First stop the diuretic. A NSAID preparation such as indomethacin should be given to con-trol pain and inflammation. Colchicine may also be used. It is given 2-hourly until the attack is controlled or diarrhoea develops. IM hydro-cortisone or ACTH should be used if oral treat-ment is not feasible. Allopurinol and uricosuric agents should be avoided for several weeks as they may precipitate further acute attacks.

347 The clinical picture is that of pseudogout (pyrophosphate arthropathy). Thus allopurinol, which acts by reducing uric acid production, is not useful. Colchicine, however, when given early is reported to relieve pain and it may be useful as maintenance therapy also. A NSAID preparation is usually the treatment of choice in pseudogout.

Soft tissue disease

348 Rapid treatment is essential in order to avoid a frozen shoulder. He should stop work for the moment. A local steroid injection is valuable and a NSAID preparation should be given also. Additional measures include ultrasound therapy and gentle passive movement.

Non-steroidal anti-inflammatory drugs

349 Indomethacin is a very effective anti-inflammatory drug, especially for night pain and morning stiffness. However, it is more likely to cause dyspepsia and peptic ulceration than are other preparations. Headache, dizziness, and depression are side effects of higher doses. Patients given indomethacin may develop retention of fluid due to a reduction of glomerular filtration rate.

350 Yes. Indomethacin and other NSAIDs reduce glomerular filtration rate and can cause fluid retention and hypertension even in normal people. This effect may be partly mediated by reduced prostaglandin production in the kidney.

Intra-articular steroids

351 From a few days to several months, with an average period of 1 month. Frequent injections may accelerate destruction of cartilage.

Neurological Disorders

Headaches and migraine

352 A patient with chronic tension headache should be helped to gain insight into his condition with a view to making changes in his lifestyle to correct any identifiable causes of stress or conflict.

353 An initial dose of ergotamine of 1–2 mg can be repeated a few times within the first few hours up to a maximum of 8 mg in any one attack.

No more than 12 mg should be taken in any one week.

Excessive intake can cause a withdrawal headache, and severe peripheral vasoconstriction with tissue necrosis. In this latter situation nifedipine is reportedly helpful.

354 Coffee, chocolate, cheese, citrus fruits, bananas and alcohol may precipitate migraine in susceptible individuals.

355 The dose of ergotamine is 1–2 mg either by SC injection or by suppository. Methysergide is particularly effective in aborting an episode of cluster headaches.

356 Lupus encephalopathy (SLE), the Guillain–Barré syndrome and cerebral sarcoidosis are indications for steroid therapy.

The benefits of steroid therapy and ACTH in multiple sclerosis are disputed.

Analgesia

357 Both morphine and pethidine can cause nausea and vomiting, particularly following IV administration. A simultaneous dose of a phenothiazine such as prochlorperazine 12.5 mg is often an effective antiemetic.

358 Codeine, which may be given in a dose of 30–60 mg every 4–6 hours. The constipation may be of therapeutic value, ensuring that no bowel movements occur during a period when straining and a rise of intracranial pressure could be dangerous.

359 Amitriptyline or fluphenazine may be effective, although it is not clear if this is a direct biochemical effect on the regenerating nerve fibres or correction of concealed depression or mood disturbance. Guanethidine has also been found effective in antihypertensive doses.

Insomnia

360 Temazepam – short-acting. Nitrazepam – medium-acting. Flurazepam – long-acting.

Epilepsy

361   The therapeutic range of phenytoin is 40–80 μmol/l. Toxicity is common just above this range due to saturation of the metabolic pathway.

362   Carbamazepine and valproic acid.

363   Valproic acid. Drowsiness and sedation are less with this drug than with other anticonvulsants. It may cause gastrointestinal upset or a mild tremor.

364   In trigeminal neuralgia it relieves pain in a significant proportion of cases.

365   Diazepam IV or clonazepam IV.

Cerebrovascular disease

366   The dose of dipyridamole is usually 75–150 mg daily in divided doses. It is a vasodilator and so may cause throbbing headaches. It potentiates the effect of warfarin.

367   In cerebral embolism. In the presence of mitral stenosis and atrial fibrillation of recent onset, failure to prevent further embolization may be catastrophic.

368   Range of movement exercises to maintain a full range of movement and prevent contractures and deformities.

Parkinsonism

369   Diphenhydramine usually brings about a prompt improvement.

370   The side effects of levodopa include nausea and vomiting, involuntary movements, postural hypotension and psychiatric side effects such as paranoia and hallucinations.

371   Bromocriptine (like dopamine) inhibits the release of prolactin by the anterior pituitary. The drug can, therefore, correct hyperprolactinaemia. It will also suppress lactation. Release

of growth hormone is inhibited, giving bromo-criptine a place in the treatment of acromegaly.

Cerebral oedema

372 The initial dose is usually 10 mg followed by 4 mg every 6 h. Following IV injection the patient may experience a tingling sensation in the lower half of the body.

Myasthenia gravis

373 Both neostigmine and pyridostigmine are taken orally. Pyridostigmine has a longer duration of action with less muscarinic effect, but its desired nicotinic effect is weaker than that of neostigmine. The daily dose of neostigmine is usually 150–300 mg and of pyridostigmine 300–1200 mg, in regularly divided doses.

Essential tremor

374 Propanolol in a dose ranging from 40 to 120 mg daily.

Narcolepsy

375 The best results are usually obtained by a combination of short, strategically placed naps and doses of dexamphetamine (or other stimulant) timed to coincide with periods of work or study. An average daily requirement would be 5 mg, three to five times throughout the day.

Infectious and Tropical Diseases

Meningitis and encephalitis

376 Penicillin G 2 megaunits IV every 2 h for 10–14 days. If the patient is allergic to penicillin or if there is doubt about the causative organism chloramphenicol 0.5–1 g IV every 6 h should be used instead.

377 Many different bacteria cause neonatal meningitis. The most important and frequent are group B β-haemolytic streptococci and *E. coli*. A combination of ampicillin and gentamicin given IV is the optimum initial therapy in most cases as both organisms should be susceptible to this combination. Further antibiotic treatment should depend on sensitivity of the organisms isolated. There is no good evidence that intrathecal or intraventricular injection of antibiotics improves prognosis in neonatal meningitis.

378 Steroids appear to be of benefit in cases with neurological defects. Some authorities use them in every case in order to try to prevent adhesions within the subarachnoid space which may lead to spinal block or hydrocephalus.

379 Vidarabine or acyclovir, both of which are given IV. The former is more toxic, causing GIT upset, neurological signs and bone marrow depression. It is also teratogenic and possibly carcinogenic. Acyclovir seems to be much less toxic. It may cause some local irritation if extravasation occurs during IV administration.

Gastrointestinal infections

380 In pseudomembranous colitis due to *Clostridium difficile*, vancomycin is the antibiotic of choice. The adult dose is 500 mg every 6 h either orally or IV.

381 Because antibiotics are not only ineffective for this condition, they may also actually prolong the illness and increase the carrier rate.

382 A short course of tetracycline for 2–3 days eliminates the vibrio from the stool and shortens the illness. Unfortunately, resistant strains have emerged recently.

383 Approximately 2–5% of typhoid cases become chronic carriers. A 6-week course of amoxycillin or a long course of co-trimoxazole terminates some of these carrier states if the gall bladder function is normal. If the gall bladder is diseased, antibiotics alone are less likely to be effective and cholecystectomy may be required. How-

ever, even this is not indicated routinely in all typhoid carriers. Chronic typhoid carriers must not work as food-handlers, and public health authorities should be informed about these patients.

384   Co-trimoxazole seems to be very effective in treating chloramphenicol-resistant cases and is less toxic than chloramphenicol. Ampicillin is also useful but probably not quite as effective as the other two drugs. With ampicillin the fever takes approximately 2 days longer to show a response.

385   This clinical picture suggests giardiasis, which is a common cause of traveller's diarrhoea. It has a relatively long incubation period, hence the development of symptoms following his return home. Treatment consists of metro-nidazole 2 g at bedtime for 3 days. Side effects include nausea, a metallic taste, dizziness and some disturbance of judgement. Thus alcohol should be avoided during therapy, and driving and operating dangerous machinery should be avoided.

Viral infections

386   The Paul–Bunnell test is indicated as this picture is very suggestive of infectious mononucleosis. A white cell count and blood film are also in-dicated and this usually reveals an atypical lymphocytosis. In most cases of infectious mononucleosis symptomatic measures only are indicated, but when pharyngeal swelling is severe, a short course of steroids usually causes rapid resolution. Vigorous exercise should be avoided until splenomegaly has resolved as there is a risk of splenic rupture.

387   First, any live vaccine is contraindicated in pregnancy. Secondly, it is contraindicated in children under 9 months due to a slight risk of encephalitis. Immunocompromised patients, including those on steroids or cytotoxic agents, should not receive this vaccine. Finally, as the vaccine contains small quantities of neomycin and polymyxin it should not be given to patients allergic to these antibiotics.

388 Diphtheria antitoxin should be given as early in
the disease as possible in order to avoid cardiovascular and neurological complications. This
antitoxin carries some risk of anaphylaxis, and
should such a reaction occur treatment with
adrenaline is necessary. Penicillin should be
given to clear the organism from the infected
area (usually the throat). Tracheostomy,
mechanical ventilation and cardiac pacing may
be necessary in complicated cases.

389 Antibiotics should not be given routinely in
established pertussis, but should be reserved for
secondary complications such as bronchopneu-
monia. Antitussives are not effective in
whooping cough. Anticonvulsants such as IV
diazepam are useful in treating fits. Sodium
valproate is useful in preventing further seizures.

390 HTIG neutralizes unbound tetanus toxin and
it should be given IM or IV as soon as tetanus
is diagnosed, and before wound debridement.
Intrathecal HTIG improves prognosis if given
early, or if the tetanus is mild.

391 Multibacillary disease should be treated with a
combination of rifampicin, clofazimine and
dapsone initially in order to prevent dapsone
resistance. Rifampicin is usually stopped after
a month, but clofazimine is continued for a
year and dapsone is continued for life if
tolerated. Treatment for life is necessary because leprosy bacilli may lie dormant in skin,
nerves or muscle indefinitely.
  Paucibacillary disease can be cured, although
3–10 years treatment with dapsone alone is
usually required.

392 Antibiotics should be given IV until clinical
improvement occurs, following which oral
therapy may be substituted. Therapy should
be continued for a minimum of 6 weeks and
frequently for 3 months.

393 In patients with sickle cell disease and following
splenectomy. In these two groups of patients
there is particular susceptibility to pneumococcal infection.

Fungal infections

394   *Pneumocystis carinii*:   co-trimoxazole
        Aspergillus fumigatus: flucytosine with am-
                                   photericin B
        Candida albicans: as for *A. fumigatus*
        Nocardia asteroides: sulphonamides in high
                                     doses.

395   Dose-related nephrotoxicity is the most serious
side effect. Thus other nephrotoxic drugs
should be avoided during amphotericin B
therapy. Other side effects include throm-
bophlebitis, fever, nausea and vomiting. The
latter may be prevented by premedicating the
patient with aspirin and diphenhydramine.

Rickettsial infections

396   The clinical and serological features described
are those of scrub typhus, a rickettsial infection
due to *Rickettsia tsutsugamushi*. This is transmitted by infective larval mites. Tetracycline is
the drug of choice, but chloramphenicol is
also very effective, although it carries a small
risk of aplastic anaemia.

397   Tetracycline and chloramphenicol are rickett-
siostatic and not rickettsiocidal. They must be
given as early as possible in the course of the
disease as they are less likely to be effective
when irreversible pathological changes have
occurred. Treatment should be continued for
48 hours after the patient becomes afebrile,
otherwise relapse may occur.

Protozoal infections

398   The major risk of toxoplasmosis in pregnancy is
congenital toxoplasmosis in the infant. In the
first trimester a pregnant woman with toxoplasmosis should be treated with sulphonamide
or spiramycin. In the second and third tri-
mesters, pyrimethamine and sulphonamides
should be used. How effective these therapies
are at preventing congenital toxoplasmosis is
uncertain.
      Immunocompromised patients are prone to
disseminated toxoplasmosis and should receive

the pyrimethamine/sulphonamide combination. The myelotoxic effect of pyrimethamine may be prevented by using folinic acid (leucovorin).

399 In areas where the prevalence of amoebic infection is low, such as Western Europe, it is reasonable to treat asymptomatic amoebic carriers. Although the disease is of low infectivity such individuals may develop acute ameobic dysentery or an amoebic liver abscess. A 10-day course of diloxanide furoate is usually effective in eradicating the infection. A test of cure (microscopic examination of three stool specimens) should be carried out 3 weeks after treatment. If cysts are still present a second course of diloxanide furoate combined with a 5-day course of metronidazole will usually eliminate the infection.

400 This picture strongly suggests hepatic amoebiasis. Ultrasound, CT or isotope scanning would confirm the presence of one or more space-occupying lesions and 90% of patients have positive serological tests. However, in situations where sophisticated investigations are not available a 5-day course of metronidazole 400–800 mg tds should be given on the basis of the clinical picture and response to this confirms the diagnosis. In addition a course of diloxanide furoate 500 mg tds, for 10 days should be given to eradicate concomitant bowel infection. Large abscesses may require needle·drainage also.

401 Local application of heat may be sufficient to clear isolated lesions (39–41 °C for 12 hours at a time daily for 1–2 weeks). More extensive lesions require treatment with a pentavalent antimony compound such as sodium stibogluconate.

402 Fever usually settles within 14 days and splenomegaly has normally regressed by the end of the 1-month course of therapy. The complement fixation test and the IgG formol-gel test revert to normal by 6 months and parasites should have been cleared from the bone marrow after 2 weeks of therapy. Failure of response is an indication for using one of the diamidine preparations such as hydroxystilbamidine isothionate.

403 Melarsoprol, an arsenic derivative, is the only drug which is of value against neurological involvement in African trypanosomiasis. However, this is a very toxic substance and itself may cause a fatal encephalopathy in addition to jaundice, diarrhoea and conjunctival injection. Also, when in solution in propylene glycol, the mixture is an irritant and may cause serious local reactions.

Malaria

404 It is important to make it clear to her that the risks of malaria, both to herself and her baby, far outweigh the risks of prophylactic drugs. There is no evidence that current prophylactic antimalarial drugs are teratogenic in the doses recommended, although if Fansidar is used in the third trimester it may cause neonatal jaundice. Therefore, if she is intent on travelling she should take 300 mg of chloroquine base weekly starting 1 week before departure and continuing for a full 4 weeks after returning. However, yellow fever vaccination (a live vaccine) is required for West Africa also. As live vaccines are contraindicated in pregnancy, and as drugs should be avoided during the first trimester, it is worth suggesting that if possible she defer her journey until after her delivery.

405 The involvement of more than 10% of red cells, and the presence of gametocytes, strongly suggest malignant tertain malaria due to *Plasmodium falciparum.* He has come from an area of known chloroquine resistance. In view of the fact that he is vomiting, parenteral therapy is required. He should be treated with IV quinine until well enough to take it orally. Tablets should be continued for 3–5 days and followed by a final dose of three Fansidar tablets (equivalent to 1500 mg sulphadoxine and 75 mg pyrimethamine).

406 The long interval between exposure and development of overt malaria, the fact that the patient was in India, and the blood changes described all suggest vivax malaria. Therapy consists of a 3-day course of chloroquine. *Plasmodium vivax* has not as yet developed chloroquine resistance. The chloroquine course

should be followed by a 2–3 weeks course of primaquine 7.5 mg bd in order to eradicate the persistent exoerythrocytic forms of the parasite. Primaquine causes haemolysis in patients with G6PD deficiency, which is especially common in blacks and some individuals from the Middle East. Screening tests for this disorder should be carried out in individuals at risk before prescribing primaquine.

407 Chloroquine resistance has not yet appeared in West Africa, but up-to-date information on resistance should be obtained from the WHO or other recognized authorities before advising patients. If he is going to continue working in West Africa he should change to another antimalarial, such as one of the antifolates (proguanil or pyrimethamine). This is because chloroquine has a cumulative toxic effect on the retina. The critical cumulative dose appears to be about 75 g, which is approximately the amount that the patient has already ingested.

Worm infestations

408 The clinical and laboratory findings indicate schistosomiasis due to *Schistosoma haematobium*. The drug of choice is metriphonate 10 mg/kg in three doses, each 2 weeks apart. It is cheap, effective, non-toxic and may be given orally.

409 Not only can this drug be used to treat individual patients with symptomatic schistosomiasis but it may also be used for mass chemotherapy in order to reduce transmission of the disease within an affected population.

410 Severe reactions to dead worms may occur, with fever, lymphangitis and abscess formation, and this discourages asymptomatic people from taking the medication.

411 The Mazzotti reaction is an allergic reaction to the death of microfilariae caused by diethylcarbamazine. Features include worsening pruritus, fever, arthralgia and aggravation of eye lesions. It may be reduced in severity by starting therapy with a small dose of diethylcarbamazine (25 mg daily) and gradually building up the full

dose of 200 mg bd. Antihistamines will reduce systemic symptoms and steroid eye drops can control the reaction in the eye.

412 The migration of the skin eruption suggests 'larva currens', and the finding of larvae in the stool indicates that this is a case of *Strongyloides stercoralis* infection. In other intestinal worm infections ova and not larvae appear in the stool. A 3-day course of thiabendazole is quite effective in eradicating the parasite. Steroids should be avoided due to the risk of precipitating an overwhelming invasive infection.

413 A long course of mebendazole appears to retard the progress of the disease, but carries the risk of side effects such as fever, alopecia, glomerulonephritis and leukopenia.

414 The boy has a hookworm infection. If this is due to *Ancylostoma duodenale* a 3-day course of bephenium hydroxynaphtoate should eradicate it. *Necator americanus* responds better to thiabendazole. The child should in addition receive a course of iron supplements.

415 Diagnosis is confirmed by finding the characteristic oval brown eggs in the stool. A single dose of piperazine citrate or levamisole will usually eradicate the infection.

416 The diagnosis is confirmed by finding the characteristic eggs of *Enterobius vermicularis* on a strip of transparent adhesive tape applied to the perianal skin at night, or by finding the adult worms in the stool. Management involves strict hygienic measures, including nail-cutting and hand-washing for the whole family. In addition, the child and any others infected should receive a single dose of piperazine citrate or a 3-day course of thiabendazole.

417 Niclosamide disintegrates segments of tapeworm and releases viable eggs. There is a possibility that these eggs may develop into larvae and migrate into the tissues of the host, causing cysticercosis. Thus it is recommended that the patient is given a purgative an hour after taking niclosamide in order to expel the eggs as quickly as possible.

418 Penicillin must be given in the first week of illness in order for it to be effective in destroying the leptospirae. After the first week symptoms are due to immunological phenomena and antibiotics will not be effective at this stage. Thus, if there is good clinical evidence of leptospirosis, penicillin should be given early following appropriate cultures but without waiting for results.

419 Parenteral penicillin G is the treatment of choice. Patients allergic to penicillin may be given IM streptomycin instead. Anthrax is rare now in developed countries due to the effectiveness of vaccination of animals and of humans who are occupationally at risk.

420 Chronic brucellosis is associated with visceral granuloma formation and responds poorly to chemotherapy. Different antibiotics have been tried, including co-trimoxazole and ampicillin, but there is no good evidence that these are any more effective than tetracycline and streptomycin.

421 All that one can offer a patient with rabies in areas without advanced medical facilities is heavy sedation and analgesia in order to control the terror and pain.

422 Firstly, active immunization is required. The vaccine of choice is human diploid cell strain vaccine (HDCSV); 1 ml should be given on days 0, 3, 7, 14, 30 and 90. Secondly, passive immunization, preferably with human rabies immunoglobulin (HRIG) is necessary to neutralize the rabies virus before the vaccine-induced antibody develops. Usually half of the dose is infiltrated around the wound and half given IM at a site distant from the vaccine site.

Sexually transmitted diseases

423 Acyclovir reduces viral shedding, healing time and duration of symptoms in genital herpes but it does not appear to prevent recurrent attacks. It may be used topically, orally or IV depending on the severity of symptoms.

424 Patients must be followed up 24 hours after therapy and 2 weeks later to confirm cure. Any residual discharge must be examined microscopically and cultured. Many strains of gonococci have recently developed penicillin resistance, which may be partial or due to production of penicillinase, in which case it is complete. Patients with initial treatment failure may be treated with spectinomycin which is penicillinase resistant. Serological tests for syphilis should be done initially and after 1 month. Treatment of sexual contacts of patients with gonorrhoea is essential, otherwise reinfection is very likely.

425 By erythromycin or oxytetracycline. The Jarisch–Herxheimer reaction is a febrile reaction to toxic material from killed spirochaetes following the first injection of penicillin. It occurs in primary syphilis and in up to 90% of cases of secondary syphilis but is less common in latent syphilis. Manifestations include fever and flu-like symptoms occurring within 12 hours of the initial penicillin injection. In neurosyphilis or cardiovascular syphilis the Jarisch–Herxheimer reaction may provoke focal lesions (cerebrovascular or coronary occlusion) and psychosis. Steroids should be given in addition to penicillin in these cases in order to lessen the reaction.

426 A 3-week course of tetracycline or erythromycin is probably necessary. Sexual contacts must be treated also. About 85% of cases respond to this, but the remaining 15% may have persistent symptoms. About 5% of cases develop Reiter's syndrome.

Drug reactions and interactions

427 Sulphonamides are inhibitors of hepatic mono-oxygenases, the enzymes which metabolize phenytoin sodium. Thus when sulphonamides are added, levels of phenytoin can rise from the therapeutic to the toxic range and produce cerebellar ataxia. Drug interactions due to enzyme inhibition tend to appear immediately, in contrast to interactions due to enzyme induction which frequently take 2–3 weeks to appear.

428   When high doses of IV benzylpenicillin are required they should be freshly prepared and injected as a bolus rather than given as an infusion. This appears to prevent formation of antigenic penicilloyl polymers of penicillin *in vitro*, and greatly reduces the risk of sensitivity reactions. A history of an anaphylactic penicillin reaction should be accepted as proof of allergy and in such cases skin testing should not be done and penicillin should not be given. However, patients with serious infections requiring penicillin, and in whom there is a less convincing history of penicillin allergy, may usefully be screened for allergy by intradermal skin testing. Even those with negative skin tests should be treated with caution and the initial test dose of penicillin should be small and closely supervised.

429   Rifampicin is one of the most powerful inducers of hepatic mono-oxygenases, which are enzymes responsible for terminating the activity of many drugs, including prednisolone. Thus the effect of prednisolone is reduced by increased metabolism of the drug. The clinical effects of a drug interaction involving enzyme induction usually take some weeks to appear. Other drugs whose effect can be inhibited by rifampicin-induced mono-oxygenases are oral contraceptives, barbiturates, quinidine and tolbutamide.

Skin Disorders

430   Specific centrally acting antipruritic drugs unfortunately are not available. H_1 antagonists are useful in some forms of urticaria. There have been some reports that H_2 antagonists benefit patients with pruritus due to systemic disease. Promethazine is one of the more useful systemic antipruritic agents but it causes drowsiness.

431   (a) Excessive bathing and the use of soap should be avoided, as this may dry and irritate the skin. Hydrocortisone ointment is effective therapy but its potency should not exceed 1% in children. If the eczema becomes infected an antibacterial/steroid ointment is useful.

    (b) Potent steroid ointments may be used

when eczema is localized and occurs in an
adult, but they should only be used for brief
periods.

432 Hormonal therapy with oral contraceptives containing 50 μg ethinyloestradiol can be effective
after about 4 months of therapy. Effectiveness
is enhanced by the addition of prednisolone
5 mg daily. Anti-androgen therapy with cyproterone acetate plus ethinyloestradiol can also
be quite useful. A new approach is to use the
vitamin A derivative 13-*cis*-retinoic acid. This
may produce dramatic improvements in about
6 weeks. Side effects include conjunctivitis,
epistaxis and hyperlipidaemia.

433 Dithranol and tar are best avoided in facial
psoriasis. Topical steroids may be used with
caution, but they may cause perioral eczema
or rosacea. The weaker preparations only
should be used, and they should be applied
only to the lesions, not to the surrounding
normal skin.

434 Etretinate is teratogenic and female patients
treated with this drug must avoid pregnancy
during therapy and for 1 year afterwards.
Other side effects include hypertriglyceridaemia,
pruritus and alopecia.

435 PUVA should be avoided as first-line therapy in
young patients and those with limited areas of
psoriasis. The main immediate risk is burning
of the skin, but there is a possible risk of skin
cancer or cataract formation in the long term.
The eyes should be shielded during treatment.

436 A gluten-free diet is indicated in all cases, even
the occasional one with a normal jejunal biopsy.
This may allow reduction or discontinuation of
the dapsone while maintaining control of the
rash.

437 It is difficult to distinguish clinically between
impetigo due to staphylococci and that due to
streptococci or a combination of both organisms. Thus Gram stain and culture is recommended in all cases if possible. This is because
streptococcal impetigo may be associated with
complications such as nephritis, scarlet fever or
erythema nodosum. Thus all cases of strepto-

coccal impetigo should be treated with systemic penicillin.

438   All close contacts should be treated at the same time, even if they do not complain of itching.

439   A severe acute attack should be managed by transfusion of fresh-frozen plasma or concentrated C1 esterase inhibitor. Intubation may be required. Further attacks may be prevented by giving maintenance therapy with attenuated androgens such as danazol or anabolic steroids such as stanozolol. These drugs are contraindicated in pregnancy.

440   Stop the offending drug. Antihistamines should be used to treat pruritus but systemic steroids may be necessary when symptoms are not controlled. One per cent phenol with calamine may be helpful as a topical preparation. The adverse reaction should be noted in the patient's chart and he should be informed of the name of the offending agent and advised to avoid it in future.

441   Corticosteroids and anabolic steroids, phenytoin, diazoxide, chlorpromazine, minoxidil and cyclosporin A may all cause increased hair growth.

Eye Disorders

442   The pupil should be kept dilated with 1% atropine eye drops. Dendritic ulcers respond to acyclovir idoxuridine ointment applied five times daily.

443   Application of an eye ointment containing an antibiotic such as tetracycline twice daily should be combined with a 2–4-week course of an oral antibiotic such as co-trimoxazole or tetracycline.

444   By diethylcarbamazine 3 mg/kg/day orally in addition to a course of steroids.

445   Firstly systemic steroids are indicated. If these fail immuno-suppression with an alkylating

agent such as cyclophosphamide or with
azathioprine is indicated.

446 This is an ocular emergency and blindness will
follow unless treatment is started rapidly. This
initially comprises 0.5% timolol eye drops
12-hourly, an IV injection of 500 mg of
acetazolamide followed by 500 mg 8-hourly
orally and 4% pilocarpine eye drops 6-hourly.
Once intraocular pressure is controlled surgical
or laser iridotomy is required.

ENT Disorders

447 By avoidance of allergens such as the house
dust mite and animal dander. Desensitization is
not very effective and antihistamines may be
of some help but tend to cause drowsiness.
Some cases respond to a nasal spray containing
sodium cromoglycate. The most effective
therapy is the topical nasal steroid beclomethasone 200 mg bd.

448 Liberal fluids plus analgesics such as paracetamol syrup or soluble aspirin should be given.
Antibiotics should generally be withheld unless
there is severe systemic illness or throat culture
reveals a haemolytic streptococcus. In these
situations the drug of choice is phenoxymethyl-
penicillin and not ampicillin. Erythromycin
may be used when there is penicillin allergy.

449 Culture and sensitivity testing of the nasal discharge is indicated. An antibiotic such as ampicillin should be administered for 5–7 days
and nasal decongestant drops such as oxy-
metazoline hydrochloride promote drainage of
the sinus. An oral decongestant such as pseudo-
ephedrine hydrochloride 60 mg 8-hourly also
assists sinus drainage. Cases which do not respond to this regime may require sinus washout
via the inferior meatus.

450 The most important measure in treatment is
thorough cleaning and removal of debris by
a skilled individual. Secondly the ear must
be kept dry, and scratching avoided. Topical
application of a steroid antibiotic–antifungal
ointment on ribbon gauze is effective in speed-
ing resolution.

451 In children under the age of 5, *Haemophilus influenzae* is the most likely infecting organism and amoxycillin is the drug of choice. In older individuals infection is often due to strepto-cocci or pneumococci and penicillin is the anti-biotic of choice.

Nutritional Disorders

Vitamins

452 Chronic intake of high doses of vitamin A may lead to hyper-vitaminosis A. Features of this condition include raised intra-cranial pressure, hepatomegaly and abnormal liver function, hypercalcaemia, alopecia and skeletal pain. The sort of doses which may lead to this picture are 10 to 20 times higher than the recommended daily allowance (750 μg of retinol daily for adults).

453 Ingestion of large amounts of vitamin C may favour the formation of oxalate stones in the urinary tract by increasing oxalate excretion and acidifying the urine.

454 Hypercalcaemia, which leads to vomiting, con-stipation, drowsiness, ectopic calcification of arteries and kidneys and renal failure. High-dose vitamin D therapy should be monitored by regular checking of the serum calcium level. However when vitamin D3 (cholecalciferol) is given in a prophylactic dosage of about 10 μg per day, such monitoring is unnecessary.

455 Water-soluble vitamin K analogues may cause haemolysis especially in G6PD deficiency and in neonates. Hyperbilirubinaemia and kernic-terus may result in the latter. Vitamin K_1 (phytomenadione) is less likely to cause these side effects and is therefore the drug of choice in suspected vitamin K deficiency. IV administ-ration of vitamin K can cause anaphylaxis, and thus the IM route is preferable.

Obesity

456 Pregnancy and severe renal, cardiovascular or

hepatic disease. Very young and elderly subjects should not undertake such strict diets. Serum uric acid rises with severe dieting and thus patients with gout should continue to take appropriate medication when dieting.

457 Patients treated with fenfluramine can be expected to lose 0.25 kg more per week than those on placebos. This effect may last for up to 5 months.

458 Sudden withdrawal of fenfluramine may cause depression and autonomic disturbances such as blurred vision and postural hypotension.

Hyperalimentation

459 Diarrhoea, abdominal pain and distension are common gastrointestinal side effects of enteral feeding. Metabolic complications include hyperglycaemia, hypokalaemia, hypocalcaemia, hypomagnesaemia and low blood levels of zinc. Minor abnormalities of liver function may also occur.

460 Strict asepsis during catheter insertion; 'catheter tunnelling', in which the cutaneous entry site is separated from the vein by a subcutaneous tunnel; careful nursing of the entry point using an iodine solution to clean the skin; avoidance of using the parenteral nutrition line for infusion of other substances such as drugs or blood; and low doses of heparin added to the infusion solution may lessen the risk of infection.

461 Patients with pre-existing hyperlipidaemic conditions and those with severe pulmonary disorders. The reason for the latter is that these solutions can decrease the pulmonary diffusion capacity temporarily. Relative contraindications include diabetes mellitus, liver disease, thrombocytopenia and coagulation disorders. Thus it would be reasonable to use a fat emulsion for a patient who has an extensive bowel resection but whose lungs are healthy. On the other hand an ICU patient with multiple system failure should probably not receive fat emulsion therapy.

462 By giving insulin which may be added to the nutrient solution or given as a continuous low-dose infusion or subcutaneously according to a sliding scale.

Poisoning and Snakebite

Poisoning/toxicology

463 Adsorbents such as activated charcoal must be given within 1 hour of ingesting the poison in order to be effective. They act by adsorbing and inactivating ingested poisons, allowing their excretion in the faeces.

464 Naloxone is a safer drug than some older narcotic antagonists which were liable to cause respiratory depression as a side effect. However, its half-life is short and patients who respond to naloxone should be watched carefully for recurrence of apnoea or CNS depression over the next 24 hours.

465 An IM injection of desferrioxamine should be given as soon as iron overdosage is confirmed and this should be followed by an IV infusion of desferrioxamine in saline or dextrose. Complications of iron poisoning requiring specific therapy include seizures, shock, acidosis, haemorrhage and electrolyte imbalance.

466 Forced alkaline diuresis should only be used when renal function is normal and a urine output of 500 ml/h with a pH of 8 should be the objective. Recent reports suggest that alkalinization alone produces almost as much salicylate excretion as forced alkaline diuresis.

467 A plasma paracetamol level of over 200 mg/ml 4 hours after an overdose of paracetamol is an indication for treatment with oral methionine or IV *N*-acetylcysteine. These act by maintaining the activity of the hepatic glutathione system which inactivates the hepatotoxic metabolites of paracetamol.

468 Phenytoin is a very useful agent in this situation.

When given IV its antiarrhythmic effect is very rapid, and it does not inhibit the positive inotropic effect of digoxin.

469 Gastric lavage should be performed if the patient is seen within hours of an intentional digoxin overdose. Haemodialysis removes digoxin from the plasma but diffusion from the extravascular pool makes this benefit short-lived. Much the largest removal (and inactivation) of digoxin can be achieved with digoxin–antibody Fab fragments.

470 Hypoxaemia and acidosis should be corrected. Ventricular tachycardia is one of the more common tachyarrhythmias seen, and it should be controlled by IV lignocaine. Immediate defibrillation may be necessary if ventricular tachycardia embarrasses cardiac output or if ventricular fibrillation occurs. Severe conduction defects are an indication for insertion of a temporary pacemaker.

471 This is the picture of organophosphorus poisoning and it demonstrates many features of cholinergic excess due to cholinesterase inhibition. These chemicals may be absorbed by inhalation and through the skin. Therapy consists of full atropinization as indicated by tachycardia and dry skin. Cholinesterase deactivation with pralidoxime should also be attempted. Diazepam is useful, especially if convulsions occur.

472 Barbiturates, non-barbiturate sedatives, salicylates and digoxin are among the more extensively studied substances which are effectively removed by charcoal haemoperfusion. Its side effects include thrombocytopenia, hypoglycaemia and hypocalcaemia.

473 Ethanol is a specific antidote for ethylene glycol and methanol. It acts as a competitive inhibitor of alcohol dehydrogenase, the enzyme which converts ethylene glycol and methanol to their toxic metabolites. An initial loading dose may be given IV or orally and it should be followed by a maintenance dose.

Metabolic acidosis usually occurs in antifreeze poisoning and it should be treated with IV bicarbonate. Haemodialysis is indicated in

severe poisoning, which is very likely after ingestion of a volume as large as 300 ml.

Snakebite

474 The main indication is evidence of systemic
effects. These are bleeding or shock. Local
swelling is also an indication for antivenom
but absence of swelling in the bitten area 2
hours after the bite excludes significant en-
venoming.

475 These measures are of no benefit and are frequently harmful, leading to greater tissue
damage. The correct first aid measures are to
apply a pressure bandage to the bitten area,
immobilize the affected limb, and transport
the patient to hospital for observation, sup-
portive measures and antivenom therapy if
indicated.

476 Antivenoms are derived from horse serum and
therefore carry a risk of anaphylaxis. They are
given IV and should a reaction occur 0.5 ml
of 1 : 1000 adrenaline should be given SC.
Oxygen and suction and ventilation equipment
must be available for immediate use. Note that
the dose of antivenom is determined by the
amount of venom injected and not by the size
of the patient. Thus the dose is the same for
children and adults.

Disorders due to Physical Agents

477 Discontinue the anaesthetic. Hyperventilate.
Administer chilled saline and dextrose solutions
IV in order to assist cooling. Promote diuresis
and provide an energy substrate. Bicarbonate
may be needed for acidosis and procainamide
for arrhythmias. However, dantrolene sodium is
the specific therapeutic agent. It stabilizes intra-
muscular calcium and causes muscular relax-
ation.

478 Close monitoring is essential as respiratory failure or circulatory collapse can occur, even
several hours after rescue. There is a risk of
chemical pneumonitis and as the water was
polluted antibiotics should be given. High doses

of steroids IV may improve survival. Fresh-water drowning may cause haemolysis which may lead to acute renal failure and hyperkal-aemia. Blood or plasma transfusions may be required for anaemia or hypoproteinaemia.

479 His clothing should be removed and his entire body surface should be thoroughly washed with soap and water in order to remove con-tamination. All radioactive materials found must be disposed of, taking care to avoid con-tamination of staff and the general public. Daily monitoring of his blood count should be carried out. He may require blood or platelet transfusions for bone marrow depression. Anti-biotics may be required if severe leucopenia de-velops. Bone marrow transplantation should be considered if severe irreversible damage occurs.

480 Coexisting hypothermia must be treated first. Then the frostbitten limbs should be rapidly rewarmed by immersion in warm water (not exceeding 44 $^\circ$C).

The feet must be protected from any trauma or bruising. Some amputation may be required for gangrenous tissue, but this should be left as long as possible as considerable recovery of tissue often occurs beneath blackened skin. A number of drugs have been shown to decrease tissue loss in animal experiments. These include intra-arterial reserpine, heparin and low mole-cular weight dextran.

481 The fluid of choice is normal saline. Dextrose is usually not required as blood glucose may al-ready be elevated due to inactivation of insulin by cold. These patients are usually hyperkal-aemic initially, and thus potassium supplements should be avoided at first but serum electrolytes must be closely followed. As many hypothermic patients have underlying infections, prophylactic antibiotics should be given.

Pregnancy and Lactation

482 Paracetamol, diazepam (except during or just before labour when CNS depression results) and ampicillin.

483 Warfarin, diazepam, carbimazole and propyl-

thiouracil, ergotamine and phenytoin all
achieve concentrations in breast milk which may
affect the baby. Isoniazid reaches the same
concentration in breast milk as in maternal
blood.

484 Once labour is established 12 units of regular
insulin can be added to a litre of 5% dextrose
in water and given over 8 hours. Blood glucose
should be monitored frequently (hourly) to
keep the blood glucose between 5 and 7 mmol/l.

485 The circulating volume is reduced in pre-
eclampsia and diuretics make this worse. Mannitol may be used for the purpose of maintaining renal function.

486 It differs with regard to the level of blood
pressure considered optimal. Reduction of
pressure to 'normal' levels for pregnancy often
causes a reduction in renal and uteroplacental
function as a result of diminished organ perfusion. The optimal level of blood pressure has
to be established for each individual by frequent measurements of serum creatinine.

487 The myometrium has adrenoreceptors and stimulation of beta receptors reduces myometrial
activity. Beta blockade should theoretically increase myometrial activity. In practice this has
not been a problem and a growing number of
reports indicate that beta blockers are safe in
pregnancy.

488 Although total phenytoin levels fall, so does
the protein-bound fraction. The concentration
of free drug (the active fraction) does not
usually change significantly. Multiple pharmacokinetic changes in pregnancy tend to balance
each other out for many drugs, as for
phenytoin.

489 If pregnancy is detected very early, the oppor-
tunity should be taken of avoiding warfarin
during the sixth to ninth weeks (when it may
cause chondrodysplasia punctata). Warfarin
should then be continued until 2 weeks before
delivery. Then heparin should be introduced,
to be stopped just before delivery but resumed
in the immediate puerperium, together with

warfarin, and continued until the warfarin effect is re-established.

490   Warfarin crosses the placenta. The maternal therapeutic blood level is toxic to the fetus because of immaturity of fetal hepatic metabolism. Heparin also causes trouble. Although it does not cross the placenta there is a significant incidence of placental separation resulting in abortion and intrauterine death.

491   Hypertransfusion with normal blood reduces the amount of HbS in the circulation and lessens the frequency and severity of vaso-occlusive and haemolytic crises. The marrow is also suppressed, thus reducing production of HbS-containing erythrocytes.

Psychiatric Disorders

Anxiety and depression

492   A beta blocker, such as propranolol, is effective in controlling the adrenergic manifestations of anxiety.

493   Tetracyclic compounds such as mianserin do not antagonize anticonvulsants or clonidine, unlike the tricyclic compounds (amitriptyline, imipramine). Tricyclics take 2–3 weeks to have an effect, whereas tetracyclics start a few days sooner.

494   Common cold remedies contain sympathomimetic amines as decongestants. When their degradation is blocked by a monoamine oxidase inhibitor, a hypertensive crisis can occur.

495   Diuretics or beta blockers. Theoretically it is preferable to use a beta blocker which does not cross the blood–brain barrier, e.g. atenolol or metoprolol.

496   Extrapyramidal disturbance is the most common side effect of phenothiazine therapy. It can be prevented by adding an atropine-like anti-Parkinsonian drug, e.g. orphenadrine.

Psychotic disorders

497 Up to 300 mg of chlorpromazine or 30 mg of haloperidol can be given initially. Subsequent doses can be varied according to the response. If this initial dose is not adequate in controlling the disturbance in behaviour, amylobarbitone sodium can be added.

498 Chlorpromazine is an alpha blocker and causes peripheral vasodilation. This may lead to hypotension and hypothermia, particularly in the elderly.

Alcoholism

499 Diazepam or chlordiazepoxide is often combined with chlormethiazole, either orally or parenterally. If restlessness is severe chlormethiazole as a continuous infusion is effective.

500 Parenteral thiamine should be continued at least until a normal diet is resumed. Doctors may unwittingly precipitate Wernicke's encephalopathy by giving glucose solutions to alcoholics who are on the verge of complete thiamine depletion.

Drug	Elimination half-life (hours)	Sampling time(s) after dose
Phenytoin	9–22 (single dose) 15–100 (chronic dosing)	Not critical
Digoxin	30–40	At least 6 hours
Theophylline	3–13	Peak (depends on formulation) Trough (pre-dose)
Procainamide	2–4	Peak (depends on formulation) Trough (pre-dose)
Lithium	7–35	12 hours after evening dose
Gentamicin Tobramycin Netilmicin	2–3 2–3 2–3	Peak: 1 hour after bolus/at end of infusion Trough (pre-dose)
Amikacin	2–3	Peak: 1 hour after bolus/at end of infusion Trough (pre-dose)

[1] When thresholds exist for both the therapeutic and toxic effects

Reproduced with permission from Mucklow, J. C. Drug levels –

of concentration is valuable[1]

Threshold for therapeutic effect	Threshold for toxic effect	Notes
None	20 mg/litre (80 μmol/litre)	Saturation kinetics, drug levels essential
0.8 μg/litre (1 nmol/litre)	Dependent on: (a) plasma electrolytes (b) thyroid function (c) PaO$_2$	Clearance dependent on renal function
5 mg/litre (28 μmol/litre)	15 mg/litre (83 μmol/litre)	Clearance dependent on hepatic function
4 mg/litre (17 μmol/litre)	10 mg/litre (43 μmol/litre)	Drug levels essential
2 mg/litre (0.3 mmol/litre)	9 mg/litre (1.3 mmol/litre)	Threshold for therapeutic effect in mania 6 mg/litre (0.8 mmol/litre)
Peak: 5 mg/litre (8 mg/litre in enterobacterial pneumonia)	Trough 2 mg/litre	Clearance dependent on renal function
Peak: 20 mg/litre	Trough 10 mg/litre Peak: 32 mg/litre	Clearance dependent on renal function

under steady-state conditions, these limits define the therapeutic range.

a clinical perspective. Medicine International, 1984: 2; 300–6.

Index

The numbers in this index are the question and answer numbers

SLE continued
   plasmapheresis 177
   pulse therapy 339
   steroids 178, 339, 356
Sleeping sickness, African 403
Slow acetylators 92
Small cell carcinoma, lung 120
Smoking, stopping 111
Snakebite 474–476
Sodium bicarbonate 196
Sodium cromoglycate
   allergic rhinitis 447
   asthma prophylaxis 101, 104
   dosage 101
   exercise-induced asthma 104
   food hypersensitivity 151
   ulcerative colitis 151
Sodium depletion 35, 267
Sodium nitroprusside 72, 73, 226
Sodium retention 131, 266
Sodium stibogluconate 401, 402
Spectinomycin 424
Sperocytosis 288
Spiramycin 398
Spirometry, incentive 123
Spironolactone 27, 29, 61, 224
Splenectomy
   haemolytic anaemia, idiopathic 291
   ITP 285
   myelofibrosis 306
   pneumococcal vaccine 393
   spherocytosis 288
   thrombotic thrombo-cytopenic purpura 287
Stanozolol 439
Staphylococcal arthritis 328, 329
Staphylococcus aureus osteomyelitis 392
Staphylococcus epidermidis 80
Status epilepticus 365
Steroids (see also specific drugs)
   acne 432
   Addison's disease 221
   allergic rhinitis 447
   alveolitis
      allergic 124
      fibrosing 125
   antirejection therapy 202, 203
   asthma 100, 104

benign intracranial hypertension 372
breast cancer 320
cerebral oedema 372
chronic active HBsAg negative hepatitis 166
chronic bronchitis 108
chronic lymphatic leukaemia 314
Crohn's disease 149
cutaneous drug reactions 440
Dressler's syndrome 81
drug-induced platelet antibodies 286
eczema 431
exophthalmos, Graves' disease 214
glomerulonephritis 175, 176, 178
gout 346
Guillain-Barré syndrome 356
haemolytic anaemia 291, 292
Hodgkin's disease 316
hypercalcaemia 254, 255
hypertension, secondary 74
hypertrichosis 441
infectious mononucleosis 386
intra-articular 351
ITP 285
Jarisch-Herxheimer reaction 425
liver disease 171
lupus encephalopathy 356
Mazzotti reaction 411
multiple sclerosis 356
myelofibrosis 306
myeloma 322
osteopenia 260
PAN 342
pneumonitis, chemical 478
polymyalgia rheumatica 343, 429
psoriasis 433
renal transplantation 202, 203
rheumatic fever 76
rheumatoid arthritis 329, 332
rifampicin, interactions with 92
sarcoidosis 122, 255, 356
side effects, avoidance 222, 260
sodium retention 266
SLE 339, 356